As NORMAL *as* POSSIBLE

A Breast Cancer Story

R. Lee Hall

iUniverse, Inc.
New York   Bloomington

As Normal as Possible
A Breast Cancer Story

Copyright © 2009 R. Lee Hall

iUniverse books may be ordered through booksellers or by contacting:

iUniverse
1663 Liberty Drive
Bloomington, IN 47403
www.iuniverse.com
1-800-Authors (1-800-288-4677)

Because of the dynamic nature of the Internet, any Web addresses or links contained in this book may have changed since publication and may no longer be valid. The views expressed in this work are solely those of the author and do not necessarily reflect the views of the publisher, and the publisher hereby disclaims any responsibility for them.

ISBN: 978-1-4401-5082-1 (pbk)
ISBN: 978-1-4401-5083-8 (cloth)
ISBN: 978-1-4401-5084-5 (ebook)

Library of Congress Control Number: 2009930579

Printed in the United States of America

iUniverse rev. date: 7/06/09

In telling this story, it is not my intent to offer medical advice, to elicit sympathy, or to make myself out to be something of a hero. I wanted to tell our experience with the dreaded disease breast cancer, and maybe offer insight and encouragement to anyone faced with a similar situation. Also, in a way, I think telling this story helps my heart heal from the devastation of her being gone.

The real hero in this story is my wife, Brenda, the beautiful person who made an impact and left an impression on everyone she had contact with, whether in a professional environment or in a personal encounter. Her legacy is evident by the sheer number of people, from all walks of life and places all around the world, many of whom I never met, who sent cards and letters of encouragement to me and had the respect and desire to attend her memorials after she was gone. She was a true friend to those who entered her life: relatives, co-workers, neighbors, and family. She never sought nor wanted to be in the spotlight; she achieved this, and when she began her battle with cancer her creed became "as normal as possible." But as many people, including me, can testify, all of her life she lived anything but a "normal" life. Sure, there are others like her, but they don't come along that often. Let me offer some examples. She went to her First Communion at about age ten with a body cast because she had broken her left arm. How? She fell out of a tree building a tree fort! At nineteen, she agreed to help build a house, telling a guy she was merely dating that she would saw boards, drive nails, climb ladders, and shovel dirt. At twenty-two she wanted a faster car to "get out of a tractor trailer's way when on the beltway." We bought a Charger with a 440 engine. By age thirty-five, she was running in freezing weather. On and on the stories can go; without a doubt she was beyond the "normal" in a good and energetic way that affected everyone she came into contact with.

Many times in this story you will see that I refer to her disease as ours, as in "our tumors, our medicines," and "we did this or that." That is because I suffered along with her, every bad scan, every new discovery, every medical decision, and every trip to the doctors and medical facilities. This was what I chose, and I never wanted it any other way. I chose to be her rock of comfort, injecting logic and hope into situations when she became overwhelmed by the sheer magnitude of them. I tried to limit the times I broke down in front of her, because each time I did so it made her feel as if she had disappointed me in some way. It gave me great pleasure, and I now think one of my greatest achievements was to have been healthy enough and strong enough emotionally to care for her until the very end. It was her desire to live until the end at home in the peaceful surroundings she had created. She never wanted the end to come in a hospital bed, with machines clicking and nurses rushing around, or maybe all alone. I was able to grant her that wish. In the end, she did not look like someone on death's doorstep. She still had good weight, color, and the faculties to understand the situation. Even on the day she passed, you would still never know by looking at her that cancer was taking her away, because you couldn't tell unless you looked at a scan or MRI.

So as you read this story—and please, feel no sorrow for her or me—take away from it a few tidbits of information and, God forbid, if you ever find yourself in this situation, maybe a little guidance. I really believe that most of us can dig inside of ourselves to find strength we never imagined we would find. I know I did. She surely had that ability, and she showed it by following the creed she set for herself in 1996, to be "as normal as possible."

Often when a celebrity gets a diagnosis of a horrific illness such as breast cancer, the attention scale will go up, as it should. But there are many, many women who are given a diagnosis of the disease that are not famous or celebrities. They are just ordinary women living ordinary lives, known to only a few hundred or so people. I wanted to convey a picture of such a person in telling this story, to express the need for all of us to never to give up trying to help in any way we can to eradicate this disease once and for all, if it is possible to do so.

It is my sincerest hope that I am able to convey the need to be involved in the treatment of this or any other medical situation that should happen to a person. You have to be or must have an advocate to insure a complete understanding of all options and care that is available for your situation. And maybe, just maybe will give added inspiration to the good research doctors and scientist to give a little more effort, explore an old idea, and take that chance to find some relief or even a cure for this dreadful and nasty disease.

Dedicated to

"Mick"

Anyone who met her was lucky;
I was the luckiest of them all.

Every story has a beginning and an end, even when the road ends with tragic loss. Our story began in 1968 when I met the sixteen-year-old who became the love of my life. I have been told to never say never, but I do not believe there can or ever will be a second love of my life.

The young girl that stole my heart was vibrant, athletic, and tomboyish in a girlie kind of way. She was immediately accepted and loved by my family, all five brothers and two sisters. She grew up in a middle-class family where she was the only female in the immediate family circle. She only had one sibling, a brother nine years her senior, so when she was nine he had already left for the military. She kind of grew up with a male cousin a few years her junior; they would build tree forts and have adventures around the woods in the area, doing things a girl doesn't usually get into. I think her adventurous spirit began at this early age.

Our first meeting wasn't planned. I was attending a teenage dance with a couple of friends, and, as with most teen dances in the late sixties, it ended with a "spotlight dance." I rarely hung around for this spectacle as I wasn't a real good dancer and wanted to avoid the embarrassment of being shoved onto the floor. As I was readying myself to leave I found that my new suede coat, the envy of many of my friends, was not on the coat rack. I began to think the worst—someone had surely stolen this valuable piece of cloth!

As I surveyed the circle of people around the "spotlight couple" I spotted my coat on the shoulders of a pretty hazel-eyed girl. She was on the other side of the circle, and as I made my way around the circle she stepped back out of the crowd just in time for me to tap her on the shoulder and tell her she was wearing my coat. She refused to give it to me, stating that a mutual friend of ours had given it to her, and it was his coat. She insisted we find this friend and get the story straight. This was a trait she would have throughout her life, honest and true to a fault! Upon finding out the coat was mine she apologized and, though embarrassed, gave it to me. Much to my surprise I got what would be the best phone call ever later that week when she called to apologize more and ask if I would be at the next dance. These dances gave us the opportunity to get to know each other because we would often sit aside from the teenage commotion and talk and laugh; boy, looking back now, I don't think anyone will ever make me that comfortable again.

After a few years of teenage dating and graduation from high school, we had already begun to talk of marriage, but we were reluctant to follow through because we felt maybe we were too young. We did not want to rent a place to live, having already witnessed the difficulties other young couples were having when rent, families, and bills seemed to get in the way of home ownership. One big influence on our thoughts and plans was my older brother who married young and in 1970 became the father of twin boys. Living in a small apartment and working as a self-employed electrician, it took many years for he and his wife to establish themselves. But I knew Mick was the one I wanted to spend my life with, as I had written on the back of my high school graduation picture, which I gave to her in 1969:

"There are some people that have a certain way of showing thoughtfulness and concern for others that make them special friends and since I found that sort of friend when you and I first met, our days together will always be like you, too special to forget." She carried this picture with her always.

As fate would have it, even though I was only twenty, I was offered an opportunity to build what would be our first home. This happened shortly before Mick's nineteenth birthday. I was ready for the adventure, but I wasn't sure how receptive she would be. I got one of the first and biggest surprises of our lifetime together when I asked this nineteen-year-old beauty to help me build a house even though we were not married and had only begun to plan a life together. She never hesitated; she just asked, "Where?" I am still amazed that a nineteen-year-old girl would say yes to a crazy idea like that. But, to my surprise, after this first one, we built four more homes for ourselves and helped build and remodel many others for relatives and friends. We never lived in a home we did not build. Many people think when you say, "build you own house" you kind of did the smaller stuff, but no, when I say we built our own house, I mean we did all the tasks associated with the construction, everything our size—we're both under five foot five—and the building codes would allow us to.

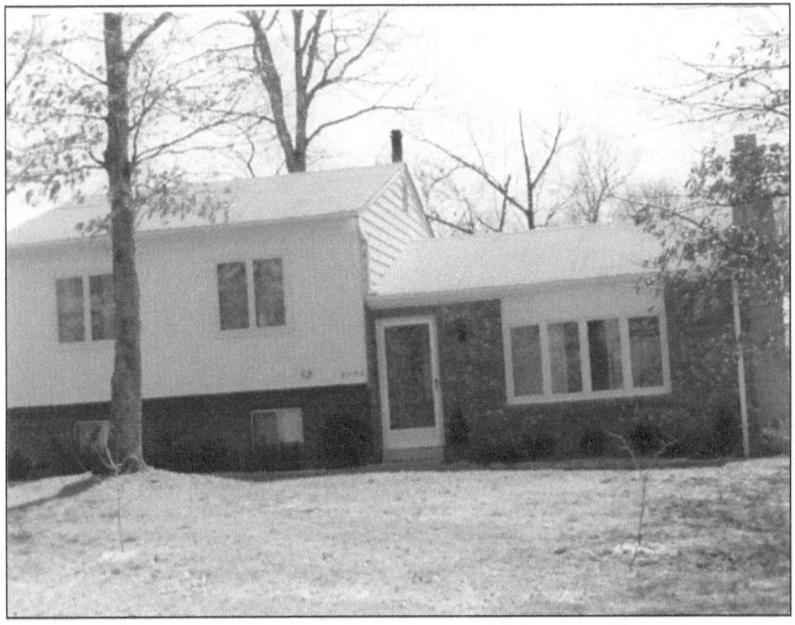

Our first house, constructed mostly by us in 1971–72

On June 17, 1972, we were married; she not quite twenty and I not quite twenty-one. She had begun working in the banking industry before we were married, and this accounting experience would be what would define a career in the federal government. I had been employed in the electrical field, and this would be where I would remain throughout my career. In the early years of our marriage I worked long hours and was away each day for twelve to fourteen hours. Although this enabled us to live comfortably and travel later, had I known our "till death do you part" was coming at an unseemingly early age, I would have spent every free minute enjoying her company and spirit.

In 1973 to keep her and I company we added to our family by getting a dog. We fell in love with a little black toy poodle, which we named Ebony. Ebony kept us company and went with us everywhere possible, the most loyal of friends. When she passed away in 1986 we vowed never to have another dog because Ebony spent most of her life alone, because of our jobs and work. But, in 1998 while living in Virginia, our neighbors brought home a dog that would become as much a part of our lives as theirs. But there was one advantage—we could send him home when we were done with him! We appreciated our neighbors for allowing us to co-own their pet, Copper. Copper has spent many "vacations" at our home in Ocean City as his "parents" travel a lot in their work!

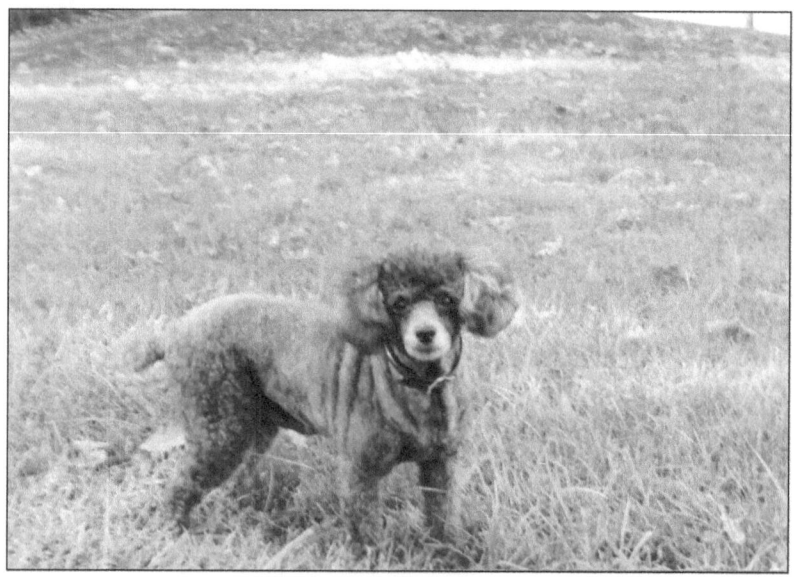

Our Ebony

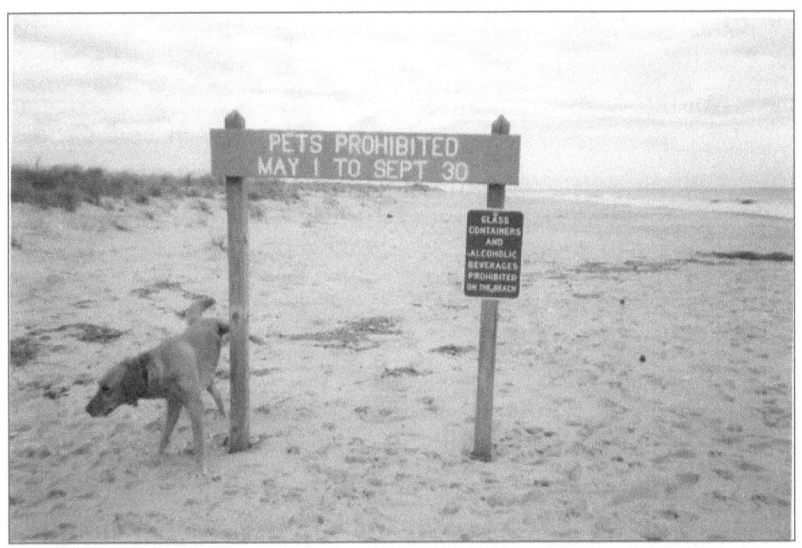

Our friend, Copper, giving his opinion of the sign

We were both athletic and enjoyed many sports: tennis, racquetball, softball, and we even tried skiing once. We always were kind of health conscious, but not health nuts. She was very competitive at all the sports we tried. She became an excellent softball player on several government office leagues, playing on all sorts of teams—women's leagues, co-ed, and, occasionally, when the men's team were short a player they would check to see if she was willing to suit up. In the late seventies during her midtwenties, she also became a dedicated runner. She started out not being able to run more than a quarter mile but gradually worked up to three to six miles a day. She would run at lunchtime or after work every day despite weather, rain, snow, ice, and even code red weather days. We spent lots of weekends at the beach, and she would run for what seemed like endless miles. Even today when I walk to the beach, there she is in my memory, running along the sand. The longest distance she ever ran was a half marathon. She would have loved to run a marathon, but after all the pounding, the knees would not stand up to 26.2 miles of more pounding.

One sport she decided to try did not last very long —rollerblading. She was very good on roller skates, but rollerblading is different in a lot of ways. On that particular weekend we were at our beach house, and she decided to go for a skate. I didn't and don't rollerblade, so I decide to ride the bike alongside her as she skated around the neighborhood. We had been skating/biking for a little while. Apparently she had gotten her nerve up and was going at a pretty good clip when she rolled past me on the bike, and I thought to myself, *this isn't good.* Ahead of us was a cut in the pavement with lots of gravel on the street. She made an attempt to turn away from the area, and, wouldn't you know it, she crashed. Going at the speed she was, I feared the worst—broken wrists, broken ankle, hurt head, all those things. But fortunately she had been wearing her wrist and knee guards, and her only injury seemed to be her pride and her butt. By the time we got back to our house her backside had turned a deep shade of purple and looked like two giant grapes. Other than the bruising she appeared to have no injuries to speak of except a couple of scrapes on her hands and legs. But in early 2008 we had an MRI of her thoracic spine that revealed an old injury to her T-6 and T-7 vertebrae. I think this was the result of that rollerblading crash, although she never complained of any back pain. The incident ended her rollerblading adventures, and she continued after this crash to be "as normal as possible."

We both had our separate careers, but we never had separate lives. It seems as though from the beginning of our relationship, until the cancer separated us, we were both content with a familiar face. As time passed and we matured I think that we always remained best friends; the one you are married to should always be your best friend. There was never a time in our relationship where I did not think, *I can't tell her this,* or that she ever felt there was anything she couldn't talk to me about. We carried this trust and bond for thirty-six years, one month, and twenty-four days, all of our married life.

I think it is sometimes unusual how we can remember with crystal clear clarity the moment we hear devastating news but not realize it as such. I think the discovery of her breast cancer is one such moment I will live with, with such clarity that it seems only yesterday.

On November 10, 1996, after her shower she came into our family room to watch television with me. She came to sit by my side and she said, "Feel this." What she wanted me to feel was a pea-sized ball, a lump under her skin about two inches above her left breast. I, the typical man, had no idea what a breast cancer tumor felt like and frankly neither did she. But we both agreed that it did not feel like something that should be there. The next few days she became anxious about the bump, and she decided to have it checked.

Inasmuch as she had been healthy and had never been to a doctor for anything other than regular checkups and a couple of emergency room visits, we did not have a family doctor. I, on the other hand, had a cardiologist and an allergy doctor. The allergy doctor entered our life after I nearly died in 1983 as I suddenly and without warning became allergic to onions and peppers. I went into anaphylactic shock—this after growing up on a farm and eating them all my life! That episode scared her so badly she was constantly vigilant about what I ate. In association with this allergy episode, I became familiar with a cardiologist to keep track of my general health. So her only thought for her care was to see her ob-gyn and get another opinion as to the process to get it checked. She made the appointment and after consultation with the ob-gyn, who recommended she have a biopsy to assure all of us that it wasn't dangerous.

On December 9 the biopsy was done. At that time, it took a few days to get results back. I went with her for the biopsy, which was done with a large needle and watched as the technicians took samples from the area around the bump and the surrounding tissue. Later that week, the doctor's office called with the results and asked her to come in and get them. We were both a little concerned when the doctor's staff stated they could not release the results over the phone. I still do not know why I was not with her when she picked up the results; it may have been that she went immediately after work to do so.

I will never forget when she walked in through the door at home. I greeted her with our usual hug and hello, and tears filled her eyes as she said, "The stupid thing's cancer." I controlled my emotions and consoled her, telling her we probably had found it early enough that it shouldn't be a problem, all the time fearing the worst because of my unfamiliarity with breast cancer. After all, here she was, only forty-four years old, and we had never thought of her having cancer in any form, especially at her age. We had both experienced the loss of someone very close due to cancer. Her father and mine had both passed away in 1990, mine from pancreatic cancer. Her father died suddenly due to lung cancer; he had never been treated for lung cancer nor were there indications he had the disease. Though she had no idea what we were about to encounter, she stated that she hoped she would be able to be "as normal as possible."

She had made an appointment to remove the bump, and the surgery would be performed on an outpatient basis at a local hospital on December 27, 1996, two days after Christmas. The required pre-op would be done on Friday, December 20, 1996. We decided it best to not tell the families beforehand so everyone could enjoy Christmas. As my wife went through the pre-op procedures, she began to cry, I think, not out of fear of the cancer, but because she had never had any type of surgery!

But I do remember her having a couple of emergency room visits at the hospital. One time occurred when we were building our third home for ourselves in Virginia in 1986 when she had to be rushed to an emergency room. We had borrowed a pickup from one of my brothers to transport some heating duct from the fabricator. This particular brother—I have five—was very meticulous about his vehicles; he kept them spotless, still does! As we were loading the duct work into the pickup bed, she closest to the cab and I at the tailgate, I asked her to let me know when to push the metal forward so as not to scratch the truck. We lifted a large piece onto the truck and I thought I heard her say okay. I pushed the metal—wrong thing to do! The metal was cradled in the inside of her left arm at the elbow, and when I pushed she jerked back, grabbed her arm, and said, "I'm cut." Not only was she cut, but also the artery was severed. She moved her hand and blood squirted about what seemed like twenty feet. A call to 911 quickly got her to an emergency room, sewed up with twenty stitches, arm wrapped like a mummy's, and disgusted as heck that she couldn't bend it! Even with the limited use of her left arm, she still continued to come to the homesite everyday after work and do whatever she could handle with one arm! But after this incident with sheet metal she never again would get near the stuff until it had been assembled. Here was a lady that could be dignified and proper with the best of them, but could hold her own in what is traditionally a man's world!

A second trip to the emergency room happened during one of her office league softball games. She played many positions, but in this particular game she was playing left field. She had begun to wear contacts; this was early on in contact technology, and she wore the hard ones. Well, this Amazon of a lady hit a high fly ball a little to the right side of left field. My wife, being as quick and agile as she was, immediately ran toward where she felt the ball would be, all the while calling, "I've got it." Apparently the center fielder didn't hear her, and leapt for the ball, just barely touching it enough to throw it off course to strike my wife in the left eye! She grabbed her eye, threw her glove, and began to bleed everywhere! Realizing that her contact was broken in a million pieces and she had a nasty gash above her eye, I rushed her to the emergency room thinking the worst—that she had lost her eyesight in her left eye! Well, the brave doctors removed all traces of the contact they could find, put eleven stitches above her eye and sent us on our way. In a few days, she had the shiner of all time—not only did she have the stitches, but the laces of the ball had left a railroad track bruise under the eye. She only missed one game.

On Friday, December 27, 1996, the day of the surgery I decided to tell one of my sisters, because everyone was curious as to why we had not spent the usual Christmas night at our relatives' home. She was upset and alarmed at first but decided she would meet us at the hospital to keep me company during the surgery. My wife was always very close to my family; my mom, dad, brothers, and sisters adopted her as one of their own from the very beginning. Mick was one of those people who had an infectious smile and attitude; you could not be around her and be mad or sad! She was the one who at my family gatherings, Christmas and holidays, would initiate the funhouse atmosphere with card games, sports activities, and getting everyone that was able involved. After we built our first beach house, everyone would stop by and visit "the funhouse." A family trait my siblings and I share is giving people nicknames, not in a vicious way but as comic relief. Some of them that come to mind are Poppins, Dumplin', Lumpy, Big Lou, Hig, Homeless Man, Geezer, Mr. Goodwrench, Mayor, Garfield, Rappin'—oh, the list could go on and on. But my wife was nicknamed "Mick" because of her affection for Michelob Lite beer, and this was the name that stuck with her. During the early years of our marriage neither one of us drank alcohol—I still don't—but sometime around 1979 two things happened. Mick had lost a lot of weight, and someone suggested beer would put some weight on her. At the same time, she began to play softball. Ever seen some of those beer bellies, or been to a ball game without beer? I remember the first time she had me buy her a six-pack for the game. She and another girl each drank three beers and got high as kites! After that, beer was a regular thing at ball games and social events, and it was pretty much always Michelob Lite. Mick also had this knack for doing crafty things, making shell wreaths, topiaries, and such, often taking two or three weeks to complete just one. She would always open a beer when she worked on her projects, saying it would help her "be creative," and I used to kid her that a particular craft would be a one six-pack or two creation. Although she was never a big fan of beer drinking outside of parties and social events, the nickname Mick stuck with her for the rest of her life.

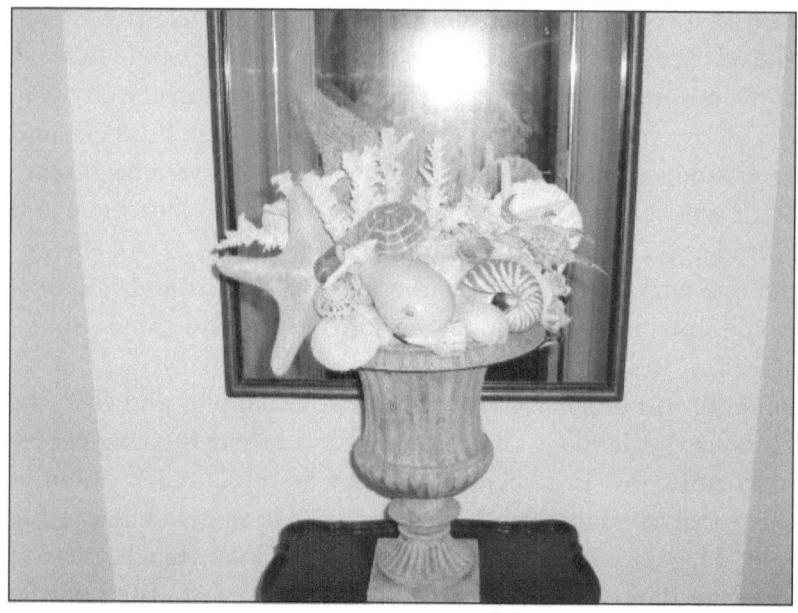

One of her "two six-pack" crafty creations, a shell topiary

The surgery took about three hours, and the surgeon, a very well-experienced doctor, but one who seemed awfully young to us, came and reported to me he had removed the pea-sized lump along with thirteen lymph nodes from under the left arm. They were sending these items to the lab for analysis, and we should have results by Monday. I, being unfamiliar with breast cancer treatment and surgery, asked why the lymph node removal? It turns out that the lymph nodes can transfer cancer cells to the bloodstream, and they can show up later (metastasis) elsewhere in the body. The lymph nodes, located throughout the body, contain many cells. They are like little intersections in the blood vessel system, and sometimes the cancer cells get into these intersections and are transported to other organs and parts of the body.

My sister and I, while waiting for my wife to be released from the recovery room, began to speculate and summarize all the scenarios where cancer could go from that point. I do not think it ever crossed our minds nor were we familiar enough to realize it could grow just about anywhere in the body; I'm sure neither of us ever imagined the brain.

After being released from the recovery room and the hospital my wife had this little drain bottle draining the incision pinned to her shirt. Although she had this little bottle and had just had surgery less than twenty-four hours before, Saturday was a very warm day for the northern Virginia area, and my wife insisted on going for a walk! She put on her walking shoes, shorts, and tights, pinned the little bottle to her sweatshirt, and proceeded to walk for about a mile. She did this each day for the next several days while the weather was warm, pinning her little bottle to her shirt and walking around the neighborhood, until soon the drain was removed and she was back to "normal." Incredible, this is the only word I can use for her wanting to get back to life as she knew it, and live up to her motto, "as normal as possible."

Little did we know this was not the end of the surgery. A couple of weeks later the doctor called and stated that the lab was not satisfied with the amount of surrounding tissue removed and wanted him to cut another "quarter inch" of border. This decision meant another outpatient surgery but under only a local anesthetic. More disappointing was that the lab stated they would not release any "preliminary" results until they examined this additional tissue.

On January 24, 1997, we reported for the next round of outpatient surgery. This was to remove more "border tissue" to allow a lab to analyze for spread of the disease. This surgery went relatively simple, but it made the first incision look small in comparison. My wife now had a two and a half inch incision across her upper shoulder area that required more stitches to close.

There was to be no recovery room time as this surgery or procedure was performed under a local anesthetic and she could go home immediately. We were informed the lab would have the results in about a week and we should call after noon about January 30 to hear the results. Looking back on this experience it now seems it was rather routine and simple, but it was a major issue for us inasmuch as my wife had never had surgery of any kind. This time the lab was satisfied that the surgeon had gotten all the area suspected of having cancer during the first surgery and the surrounding tissue removed on January 24 was "cancer cell free."

SISTER REMEMBERS

When I began writing this story I thought it would be interesting to have input from other family members about the impact my wife had upon them. Most of them thought it too emotional to put pen to paper, but my baby sister, Jane, did want her thoughts to be included in this story. This chapter is her story.

When my sister-in-law first appeared in my life, I was the ripe old age of twelve, going through my own emotional and physical steps of puberty. She was everything I longed to be. She had all the cute clothes and the popular friends, and she was very cute. I wanted to be just like her, so imagine how thrilled I was when she decided to start giving me her "old" clothes. I was then part of the cool clique at Eugene Burroughs Junior High School. I would watch her moves and style, hoping to pick up on some small detail that would make me just as cool.

My, how times change. From that young girl, I grew into a woman who respected Mick in a whole new way. You see, all of those things that I thought were so important to strive for and become really meant nothing. My sister-in-law used to laugh at me when I told her I wanted to be just like her; she never understood why. She never thought there was anything special about her. How wrong she was.

The times began to change when we were both in our twenties. My brothers were into drag racing, and she and I started going to the track. We would whoop and holler and drink our Mick beer. When we left the track it was usually late and Mick and Ray would often stay at our home. We'd sit up and talk until three in the morning. Don't worry, my brother was always there to make sure we were safe; he never drank, and when we got home, he would just kiss her good night and off the bed he'd go. Meanwhile, she and I would be planning our next adventure. I think that's when we got into the world of flea markets and antiques.

15

Mick's heritage is from a small province in Germany called Silesia. This area of Germany had many porcelain factories, and it was rumored one of her ancestors owned one with the marking C. Tielsch. We started our hunt for porcelain with the Silesia marking, and I think at one time we must have thought we owned most of the pieces on the east coast. Once we had our fill of Silesia porcelain, she started looking at old lace and antique mirrors, and of course I followed right along in her footsteps. Both our jobs required that we travel, so we always looked out for one another's interest. We couldn't wait to tell each other about our finds.

After the old lace and antique mirrors, we moved on to different areas. I loved songbirds, Santa Claus, and anything Christmas. She continued pursing her love of nautical items; she loved seashells. We hit every antique flea market on the east coast, but our favorite was Brimfield, which we began to make a regular trip in the midnineties. I had a motor home, and we'd hop in and drive all the way there from Maryland. It was great because we could park the motor home in the field at the flea market so we had a place to come and eat or rest or have a Mick. I can still see the excitement in her eyes when she discovered her treasures—old prints of sea life, plates with hand-painted shells. She usually had a plan to decorate with her finds.

My sister-in -law hated secrets. I remember one year I found one of those huge clam shells that weighs about seven hundred pounds in someone's front yard. Well, seeing a chance to give her the perfect Christmas gift, I left a note on the door of the home informing them I'd like to buy the shell if they were interested in selling it. They were, and I did. After I got my brother to help me bring it home to our garage, it stayed there from August until Christmas of that year. I had to keep her out of the garage most of the time so she, as curious as she was, would not say, "What's under the blanket?" I teased her all the way up to Christmas. Once Christmas arrived, I left all these different clues throughout the house so that she had to complete a treasure hunt to find her prize. When she finally reached that big shell, she was thrilled, and tears of joy filled her eyes. She couldn't wait for me to tell her where I got it. I think that gift meant more to her than anything I had given her before or since.

I mentioned that I traveled a lot in my work. Well, anytime I planned a business trip, I always called to tell her and report the destination so that she and my brother could decide if they wanted to tag along. They often did, and each trip we ended up having some great treasure hunting adventures.

When I first learned of her cancer, it was sort of a surreal feeling for me. I kept thinking, *Oh, it's not that bad. They got it in time; she's strong and healthy.* But I remember going to the hospital with my brother when they removed the lump above her breast and lymph nodes from under her left arm. Seeing her go through that painful treatment, still managing to keep a smile on her face, was amazing. She always seemed to weather each storm well. Then, the cancer disappeared for years, or so we thought.

Although I have seven siblings, for some reason, I became closely attached to Ray. When he asked me to put down a few words about my sister-in-law, his wife, I didn't think I could do her justice without describing him as well. He is one of the most caring individuals you could ever meet, but he has a few qualities that are very unique. The one of which I'm most fond of is his ability to listen. No matter what the situation, no matter if he feels you are wrong or right, he always tries to see the other side and get you to focus on the big picture. His ability to communicate through his words, whether in the form of a poem or just sitting on a porch talking to you, is something I will always treasure. She was very similar to him in this fashion, although she was not as patient; perhaps she had a reason for her impatience.

My sister-in-law loved the sun, the beach, and the outdoors, and she also valued her friends and family. She was the type who never had to look for friends; friends found her. She was never an in-law to me—she was my sister. I came to realize that looking up to her wasn't what it was all about—growing up with her meant so much more, and I'll treasure those memories. During the last weeks of her life I had a conversation with her, and she asked, "Are you happy, Dumplin'? Just please be careful, I will miss you." I will never forget those words, her facing all that she was and worrying about whether I was happy.

When she and I traveled, we never knew where the antique stores were in the area, so I began to tear out the "antiques" page of yellow pages and off we'd go with our listing and our map. When I first did this, she thought it was terrible. "What if the next people needed those pages?" she'd ask.

"Come on," I would say, "How many people even look at the phone directory when they are in the hotel room, much less need the pages that contain antiques?" Every trip she made after that, there were a lot of hotel rooms with a page or two missing from the yellow pages. I heard later she had even conned co-workers into bringing back those pages from the directories where they traveled.

Another fond memory I recall was when she and I were in Pennsylvania at a flea market where found these two old pictures of a man and woman that appeared to be from the days of George Washington. Neither of us cared for the people in the picture; we only wanted the old gold gilded frames they were in. So, upon returning to the hotel, we quickly discarded the old people in the trash outside our room, keeping our prized frame. We joked and laughed about how we'd wake up the next morning to find "George and Martha" at the door. Well, when we woke up the next morning, the pictures of George and Martha were leaning against the trash bin staring directly at our door. We got a good laugh out of that, and even joked we probably shouldn't have discarded them in that manner!

When it came to eating fried chicken Mick had no equal at cleaning the bone; she could clean a piece of chicken like there was no tomorrow. She ate everything off of it, seemingly all the way down to the marrow. She would not allow us to leave meat on the bone of a piece of chicken; we never threw "good bones" away because we knew she would come along and savor any remaining morsels. I remember when she and Ray were building their home in Virginia, my brother had left a carryout box containing the remnants of his lunch sitting on some lumber in the garage. Every day after work she would show up to help build the home and she would always check for "snacks." She arrived and headed for the chicken box. After she finished cleaning the bones, my brother asked if she was hungry, and she said no because she just finished his chicken. He asked, "What chicken?" Then he convinced her that the box was not his. The look on her face was priceless because she thought she had eaten a stranger's leftovers. Neither of us could contain our laughter, and we had to admit to her the leftover chicken bones were his.

My sister-in-law never cooked too much, boy, that's an understatement, although she was usually the first one to want to be of help in the kitchen. Sunday dinners were often spent at the family home, and on their way home from the beach they would often stop for Sunday dinner. This particular time she decided she would do the mashed potatoes, by the time she had finished the "mashed potatoes" they were a little thin, so thin as a matter of fact we used them for gravy over our meal. There are so many memories and stories about "Mick" I could go on and on.

=== GONE TOO SOON ===

Like the sunset disappearing with the rising of the moon
like the fading colors when you release a bright balloon
like a shooting star going across the evening sky
like a rainbow that vanishes before your eye
like a castle built upon that sandy beach
like one step further, that's beyond your reach
like the birds I wait patiently to hear sing
like the anticipation an antique venture brings
like the snowflake you follow until it hits the ground
Like a joyful memory you've suddenly found
like trips through fields searching for shells and lace
like the vision I have of your smile, your face
like a chapter of my life, pages torn away
With these verses I write, you're in my heart to stay
like a favorite old song, and you hear the tune
like all of these thoughts, you are gone too soon.
this loving memory will help my brother's way
Don't forget to remember, she's in his heart to stay
their souls are forever intertwined
memories are the gift she's left behind
after all we'll remember she's back where she began
back in heaven, resting in God's hands.

My sister Jane wrote this poem after my wife's passing.

As instructed, we called back two days after Mick's second procedure, with great anticipation as to the results from the lab. Our first diagnosis was confirmed; the lump was breast cancer, but there more devastating news. Along with the positive confirmation that it was breast cancer, we also were told that of the fifteen lymph nodes removed at the time of surgery, three were positive for cancer cells. This, they told us, would greatly affect the choices we made and direction of treatment protocol.

Affect the treatment protocol? How about affect your life? Here it was coming on to the spring and summer of 1997, and Mick was so looking forward to another summer of flea markets and antiques, getting back to running, weekends at the beach, and more work-related travel. Since early in our relationship Saturdays and then weekends at the beach. When we were dating we could load up the car early in the morning on Saturday, drive to Ocean City, spend a day relaxing on a part of the beach in north Ocean City which in the late sixties was kind of deserted, then head home and be there by nine or ten in the evening. People used to ask us, "Why do you want to be up there; there's nothing there?" That was our point—nothing there meant we were away from the crowds and noise so we could enjoy each other's company and continue to fall in love. We both had affection for the sea, waves, and water that never went away all through our married life. In the late seventies, after a little bumpy time in our relationship, we decide to begin traveling to beach places—islands in the Caribbean, Mexico, and Bermuda. We saved our money and began to go two times a year, once in spring after peak season and once in the fall right before peak season. I think she had two favorite islands: Bermuda, which she would visit two additional times on work-related stuff in the late eighties, and St. Thomas—yeah, shopping! Another of our favorites was Eluthera, in the Bahamas. We visited at a time before it was so commercialized;

when for miles and miles you and your companion were the only ones on the beach.

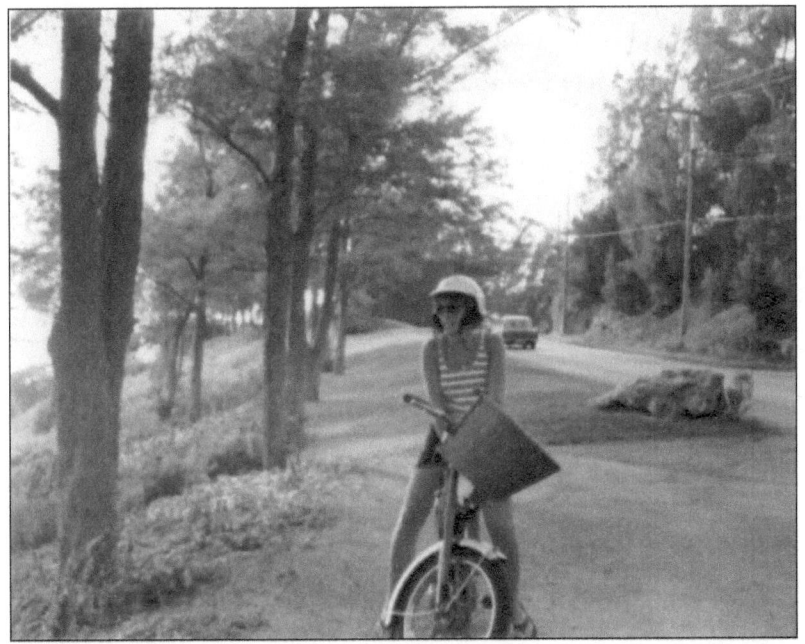

Scooter riding in Bermuda

Thinking about Bermuda brings back a fond memory of Mick and her desire to have her favorite beer, Michelob Lite, on a Sunday in Bermuda. At the time we were visiting in the early eighties, Sunday sales of packaged beer were illegal. She wasn't one to go and sit at a bar and have a beer or two, plus she wanted to go to the beach that afternoon. We were cruising around St. George's and stopped at a small store and told the clerk of her desire. Well, the ordeal turned into something from a James Bond movie. He told of a bar across the street and gave us the name of a guy to ask for, but first we had to go to the back door and knock three times; this was the signal to show we had been sent by this individual. We did as instructed and a little man who looked like a lost pirate came to the door and quickly whisked us inside and asked what kind of beverage we wanted. My wife expressed her fondness for the Mick Lite; with that, he went into the cooler and packaged her a six-pack in a dark paper sack so no one could detect its contents. Then he told us it would be twenty U.S. dollars. I swallowed hard and paid the twenty and away we went with her beer strapped to the back of my scooter. I often teased her that this was the world's most expensive six-pack, so she should enjoy each sip. She did; the beer lasted for three trips to the beach.

Inasmuch as the lymph nodes were positive for cancer, we were told the pros and cons of different treatment regimens. First, the doctors involved all strongly agreed that radiation of the tumor area was a must, and there should be no discussion about that. Everyone thought it best to delay radiation until after chemotherapy was completed. Then came the topic of chemotherapy and the various options and which would be of the most benefit for my wife's situation. The doctors explained to us that there were several chemo drugs, intravenous ones, and it was a matter of what would be the accepted treatment for this situation. At this time doctors were treating breast cancer as kind of a one-size-fits-all, but luckily as time progressed and as our subsequent battles went on, the doctors began to treat each case as an individual one, and there were some important differences offered in treatment regimens.

The first treatment regimen was to do the chemotherapy, and the final choice among the doctors was a drug called adriamycian, along with cytoxian. These two drugs were to be administered intravenously in a slow drip fashion. There would be four treatments one each month beginning on February 14, 1997. We had the choice of when and what days of the week. My wife chose to have the treatments on a Friday afternoon so that if there were side effects, she could recover by Monday and be back at work, continuing her desire to be as normal as possible

We set out for her first treatment not knowing what to expect. We took along a small snack and a couple of movies for the DVD player at the facility. When we arrived at the office, there were other women there with tubes running into their arms from the drip bottles of the various cancer medicines. There were big comfortable recliners and juice and water available for those that desired it. My wife took her chair; the nurses inserted a port in her left arm, set up a bag with a color of orange Kool-aid, and turned the valve. So began our experience with chemotherapy.

After the first treatment, which lasted about three hours, we went home expecting a volatile night. As it turned out, they always give a prescription for nausea because many women get violently ill when given chemo, which is really a poison to our body. Our fears of a fitful night were not realized, as my wife seemed to tolerate the chemo well. As a matter of fact, as the treatment went on, the nurses remarked that she should become a poster lady for the treatment! There were a total of four of these Friday afternoon treatments, after which she would crash for a couple of days, very tired and sometimes so much so I carried her to and from the bedroom. Even though these treatments made her very weak, by the third one she wanted to get to the beach to relax and recover at our beach home. Whenever we went there she seem to be in better spirits and her energy level always picked up. But, without fail, by Monday morning after each of these treatments she would be up and about and ready to return to her office and get back to normal, for it was always her intent and desire to be as normal as possible.

At this time protocol in breast cancer treatment was to administer a drug called tamoxifen. This drug was at the time one of the most advanced solutions medical people had to prevent reoccurrence of breast cancer, having proven very effective in clinical trials. This drug was in the form of a pill which was to be taken every day for five years after the initial diagnosis. My wife went along with this routine, a pill every day, but after two and a half years the side effects took their toll on her—tiredness, extreme hot flashes, endometriosis, memory loss, and a chance of other cancers are some of the many—so she decided to stop taking the tamoxifen. The doctors all had strong feelings about this and tried to encourage her to follow the standard protocol. Looking back now, was this a fatal decision on our part? Would there have ever been a reoccurrence if she had continued to take this medication as prescribed? We knew of others who had taken the tamoxifen for the recommended five years; some had taken it for as many as seven years, and as far as we knew none of these ladies had suffered a reoccurrence. She and I talked about this when the reoccurrence did in fact happen. To our credit, we did not dwell on it as a major factor in looking for a cause for any reoccurrences. We lived with the decision we had made, and this is what you must do when you need to focus and go with the here and now.

Then came time to do radiation therapy to the area where the tumor had been located. This procedure required "set-up" which involved determining the area to be radiated and the dosage to be given. To mark the area my wife was tattooed with several permanent ink dots to mark the perimeters of the area. This was a procedural requirement to assure the radiation was contained in the desired area each time treatment was administered. The radiation treatments began on June 10, 1997, and were done every weekday until July 28 of 1997. After the initial set-up appointment the treatment only lasted for about forty-five seconds under the machine. It was a relatively quick and painless process, more a nuisance that she had to go everyday after work to stare at the big machine.

Of course, it has become common knowledge in cancer treatment that with these drugs and radiation treatment they always say, "you may lose your hair." Well, inasmuch as I have learned and now have the benefit of hindsight, there is a 99 percent chance that you will lose some or all of your hair! Mick's hair loss began shortly after the chemotherapy had finished, about halfway through the radiation treatment. It was just a little hair loss at first, then clumps of hair at a time. This experience was particularly demoralizing and depressing to my wife as she had finally grown her hair back to almost the length it was at her high school graduation, some twenty-six years earlier.

Every morning she would get up to shower for work and look down and see masses of hair going down the drain. Disappointment and depression would set in. I watched in anguish this morning ritual for about a week. It had as much hurt for me as her, not so much the fact of her hair loss, but her sadness. I then took it upon myself to get her father's old hair clippers. He had kept them for many years—a strange keepsake, as he was bald. I did not mention this to her for fear it would send her into a more depressed mood. But, after several mornings of watching her tears I told her, "I can end the depression you are feeling each morning as you watch your hair falling out." I asked her, "Can I just cut it all off?" To my surprise, she said if we had clippers she would do it right then. I told her about having her dad's set.

Her haircut began with a hug and assurance from me that I wasn't in love with her hair. She then kissed me and said, "Let's do it." I assured her I had cut hair before, a little white lie, as I had never done so much as trim anyone's hair before. I just figured if I were cutting it all off, there would be none left to say I had done a bad job! We sat her in a bar stool outside on our porch and as I proceeded to give her a buzz cut any marine recruiter would be proud of, we would stop at different points as the hair was cut off and laugh about the way it looked.

After she got over the chillness of having no hair, we breached the subject of a wig. She wasn't sure this was the route she wanted to take, but she did say if she got one it would be real, meaning real human hair. Since this was a Saturday, we went to the local mall and found a wig store that did in fact have the capability to order a natural human hair wig. She tried on many different styles and colors; this was the first time I had seen her laugh that hard in quiet a while. She tried on every thing from Dolly Parton style to pageboys to afros. In the end she selected one that was as natural as could be, a perfect match to what she had just lost.

We waited about a week for the wig to arrive. In the meantime she started to use her running scarves as a cover for around the house and during her running routine. Remember, this is a dedicated runner, and even during the chemo treatment she had continued to run or walk every day except the Saturdays and Sundays after treatment.

We also went to stores where she began to select hats of all sorts to wear to work and other places we would go. She found a blue denim hat, which became her favorite then and during the next battles with this disease. Well, the "real hair" wig arrived, but as I could have guessed, she didn't like it. She said it had "too much hair." We learned that there were people who thinned wigs and hairpieces, and there was one locally at a shopping mall near us. We decided the wig was too expensive to give up on, so Mick decided to see what a thinning would do. The people at the shop were very receptive and talented at what they do. After what seemed like two hours, Mick agreed that it was so natural and close to her real hair that it was difficult to tell she had a wig on her head.

We left the mall her with her wig, and I was proud to have satisfied her desire for a "real hair" wig. But our joy was short-lived. We had driven about ten miles when she suddenly pulled the wig from her head, dropped it into a shopping bag, and proceeded to tie her favorite scarf back around her head. I just stared for a minute or two and then managed to ask, "What's wrong with it now?" Her reply made me proud and amazed that she would forgo any wigs or hairpieces through this and subsequent cancer battles.

She said, "It's too hot, and I feel like a fake." The next week she donated the wig to a local cancer center. But even after this episode there was to be another wig purchase; more about that later.

July 28, 1997, was an especially good day for us. It was the last day of radiation, the chemo treatments were over, and we were happy to have survived them without a great deal of complications; remember, doctors teased her about being their poster lady for the treatment. In our minds this meant just routine checks after this, so we could get back to normal, even though she had not strayed far from "normal" during this whole ordeal. We had continued our weekends at the beach, and she had also begun some work-related travel again, so our recovery was well on the way.

I am a firm believer that diet and attitude play an enormous role in recovery and how we respond to the issues relating to any illness. I had no doubt about my wife's attitude; it was always positive, with the firm belief she could beat the cancer. Even after the return of the disease in 2005 she wrote in her diary, "I'm going to beat this and live some long years to enjoy retirement with the love of my life."

As far as diet was concerned, I took to my role as nutritionist and chef. I had always been the cook of note in our relationship. Oh, she could cook, she just didn't like to. As a matter of fact, an invention that brought her elation as far as the kitchen was concerned was—the microwave! I remember when we were dating and she was, oh, maybe seventeen. One day we borrowed my brother-in-law's boat and, along with my brother and his wife, rode down the bay, found a little secluded place, and proceeded to have a picnic. Mick was in charge of grilling the burgers, and everything went well, except that she forgot to flatten the meatballs into burgers. Instead we had these huge meatballs grilled to perfection.

We quickly learned that chemo and radiation destroy healthy cells along with the cancer cells, and one way to counteract the death of the good cells was to increase Mick's intake of foods rich in protein. I am not saying this will or should be the case for everyone, but for her it seemed to keep her strength up, and she experienced very little side effects or weight loss during this ordeal. As part of my help in her recovery, I prepared foods rich in protein: red meat, even though we had not been meat eaters; green veggies; lots of fish—tuna steaks, striped bass (rockfish), pure Alaskan salmon—and even though she had always been a water drinker, I encouraged her to drink more water. The drinking of the water may have, in fact, helped her to flush the chemo and meds through her system relatively quickly.

By late August of 1997 she actually got a big thrill when she realized her hair was returning, slightly at first. Then it seemed like overnight she had the cutest full head of curly, dark black hair! She had never had curly or black hair before, nor had her hair been extremely thick. This was another boost to her belief that she had maybe in fact survived this bout with this ugly disease. Her hair continued to grow at an amazing rate and it continued to be curly and black! She was so proud to have hair again that she even put away all her scarves and hats.

Her recovery hit a setback in early 1998. It wasn't an issue with her health but that of a relative. Her first cousin, one year her junior, was given a diagnosis of breast cancer, but hers was in a later stage; it had already spread to other parts of her body. The reason the diagnosis was so late was that the cousin had been caring for her mother and thought her back and neck issues had to do with assisting her mother. She actually went to get examined when she thought she had injured herself assisting her mother. This was a big hit to my wife's recovery as she was close to this cousin, having grown up with her, and we feared the worst. But being the person she was, my wife then forgot about the concerns she had and the battle she had just been through. She offered words of encouragement and positive thoughts about treatment and the side effects of each thing she had been through about a year earlier. I think my wife's encouragement gave a sense of hope to her cousin, helping her believe that each day is a new start.

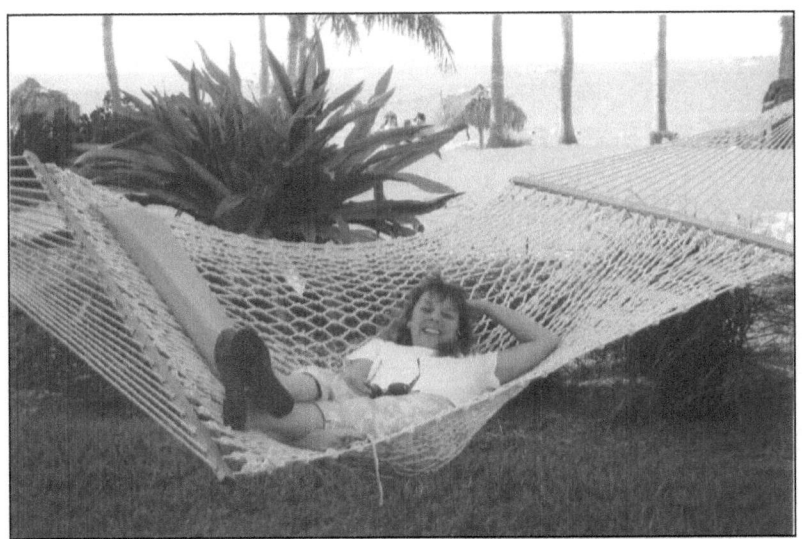

Mick's cousin on some beach somewhere

The recovery period included regular visits to the doctors; monthly at first, then every three months, and by late 1999 the doctors gave her the good news that she had to visit only every six months. By early 2000, my wife was the picture of health. She still was run/walking, and she had bought a treadmill and free weights to keep her healthy through the winter months. Although she bought this equipment and exercised regularly she wasn't by any means a physical fitness nut.

That year my bother and his wife decided to build a new home at the beach on a lot they had owned for many years. Being the experienced homebuilders we were, my wife and I offered to help. She had recovered to the point that she had no fear of doing any job—framing, plumbing, electrical, roofing, whatever was in store for the day, she was there at the ready. Never in her imagination did she use the "C" word as an excuse for not being able to do anything! This home construction began in early May and that week was to be our annual trip to Brimfield for the flea markets. As we packed up the site that Tuesday evening, saying good-bye to my brother, we backed out of the drive, and she looked at me and said, "I can't leave them like this." We had only been working on the home for four days and we still were not under roof. She chose to stay and get the home under roof, saying there would always be another Brimfield. This was the way she was, always wanting to be helpful and not to leave anyone in a bind, sometimes even giving up her own plans to help. To this day my brother and his wife chuckle about her telling us she could put the roof shingles on, but she did not like being close to the edge. In order to help her overcome her fear, we set up a scaffold she could use until she was a few rows of shingles up the roof. That way she would not be close to the edge. After a few minutes, apparently the first time she had to move the scaffold, we saw her leg dangling from the roof. We went to see if she was okay and found that she had discovered she wasn't that afraid of being close to the edge after all and it was much easier to slide along rather than move the scaffold! I tell you this just for encouragement and to show life does in fact return to normal after a battle with cancer. I think that my wife's attitude of being as normal as possible was also a lifestyle she lived.

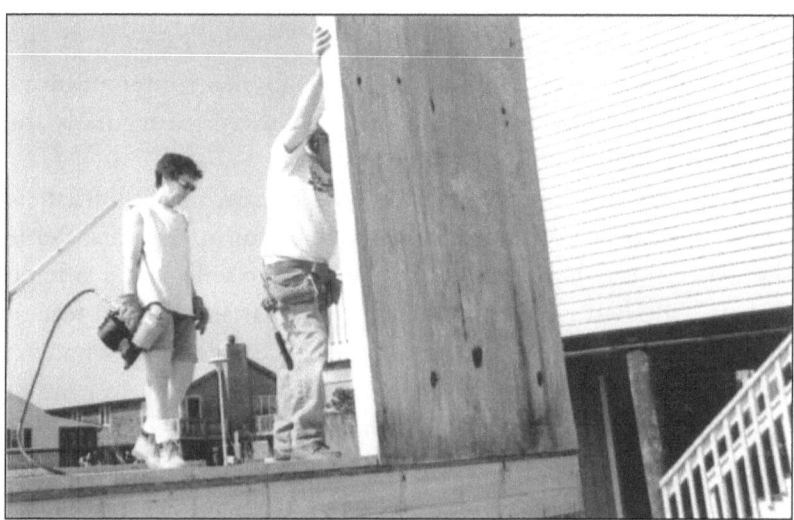

**This was the beginning of my brother's house,
May 2000, after Mick's first battle.**

As I look back at her recovery time and subsequent doctor's checkups, I wish we had known more and been more aggressive in her care. There might have been an outside chance we could have changed the course of the reoccurrence by more scans, CTs, and MRIs. Some doctors are reluctant to order scans, MRIs, and such if there are no outward signs of the disease, but as a patient I think you have every right to request these procedures. We followed the normal protocol and had faith in the doctors, who were all very good, but if given the chance we would have insisted on regular examination through the use of all of the above, especially given the situation of the positive lymph nodes. I like to refer to her checkups as the three "p's"—push, pull, and poke. The doctors would push on her feet and arms, have her pull on their hands or arms, and they would poke at her stomach and abdomen.

She became so accustomed to their procedures she would have fun with them. When they would tell her to touch her nose she instead playfully touched theirs; when she would pull on their arms or hands, she always put a little extra into it. I don't think she ever looked forward to a doctor's appointment, but she learned to accept them as part of the life we had been given. It was "normal," given her situation, to have to endure them.

From early 1998 through late 2001 our lives were much back to normal. Mick's job required travel around the world, and she had missed that during her treatment regimen. But she was soon back to traveling, and I as always tagged along whenever I could. One particular trip I remember was in 2001, when she had to go to Key West Naval Air Station—yeah, tough assignment, huh?—for some contract work. I, along with my sister-in-law, decided to take a week off and go with her. Upon arriving at the Key West airport, I went to get our rental car and the clerk asked normal chitchat about our reason for visiting. My sister-in-law and I replied we were there for vacation and pointed to my wife and said, "She has to work," to which the clerk replied, "Oh, what kind of work does your daughter do?" Well, after we told my wife this, she gloated all week long and kept referring to us as Mom and Dad. She felt especially good that someone would think that; after all, she had just had her first bout with cancer and treatments and she was probably feeling a bit old.

Then, as luck or fate would have it, the next health issue was mine. A couple of weeks before Christmas of 2001 I began to feel sluggish and out of sorts. I did not immediately seek medical help, but on New Year's Day, 2002, I had to go to an emergency room because I thought I was having a stroke. Since this story isn't about me, long story short, it turned out the nerves sending signals to my heart had a mind of their own. I wound up at age fifty having to have a pacemaker installed to regulate several functions concerning my heart.

Although I wasn't too concerned about my heart and my serious food allergies, Mick was concerned to the very end. Unbeknownst to me—and I did not find out until her memorials—she had contacted several people, relatives and friends, and asked them to look after me when she was gone. About a year prior to her passing, I had had another anaphylactic shock episode, and it scared her again badly. I think this episode weighed heavily on her mind. She apparently had contacted them in March after we heard the word "terminal" attached to our situation. My future and well-being would be a topic of several of our "hard talks" as time grew short. Here she was, facing her own mortality, and her date with destiny, but still fretting about me—you see, this was her being as normal as possible. Maybe that's why with her last words she said to me, "You're gonna be okay."

So, after the ordeal of getting me straight again, with the help of a pacemaker, our lives continued to go on without any health issues, just regular checkups and such. But then, in November of 2002 she discovered another bump in roughly the same area as the first surgery. At first we thought this to be scar tissue but, after we consulted with the surgeon who did the first surgery, he said it would be best to biopsy again just to be sure there wasn't another cancerous tumor. He removed a piece of tissue, 3.8x2.2x1.5 cm, and sent it to the lab to be analyzed. We were happy to hear the next day that this specimen was negative for any malignancy.

This episode taught us to be even more vigilant about checking for "bumps" and tissue that just did not feel right. So another scary episode came about in September of 2004, this time with another spot that just did not feel like it belonged where it was. Back to the surgeon again, another tissue removal, another lab test, and again, elation. This sample also was proven to be benign tissue with fibrosis. Again, we were happy to have erred on the side of caution; although now so much tissue had been removed from the area she had an indentation above her left breast.

I want to answer a question you might be asking at this point: "Why not a full mastectomy of the left breast?" The answer to that question lies in what the doctors, three of them specialists, had told us. Their feelings were that, since the original tumor and subsequent masses were not actually in the breast, they saw no need to completely remove the left breast. There were no indications of masses or anything indicating the cancer cells had infiltrated the actual breast. Actual mammograms, CTs and MRIs of her breast had never indicated anything abnormal in the breast tissue. These were perfectly good observations to us because we could clearly see the incisions and tissues removals were all concentrated about two and a half inches above her left breast. It also gave her a much more comfortable feeling knowing this was their line of thinking. She had even suggested it might be better to remove the suspected breast. She did not object at all to having a complete mastectomy to, "get rid of the fear, once and for all," as she put it. And, as fate would have it, we were proven correct in our decision not to remove the breast; the reoccurrence probably would not have been prevented by the mastectomy.

It had long been a dream of ours to retire early from our jobs and enjoy each other and do whatever we felt like on any given day. Early on it our marriage she had been in charge of money and finances; it was only natural, since after all, she did work at a bank! But after about two years of marriage I could no longer watch her stress over financial issues. Even though we were far from being rich, we struggled and managed our mortgage and bills. Remember, we built our home in 1972, and our mortgage was—get this—$232.40 a month! But, let's put this in perspective; she was making—ready?—$6,500.00 a year! Along with my salary of about $12,000, we were getting by. Because of her stress level, I volunteered to handle the finances until she wanted to do the job again. She never did want the job back! Throughout the rest of our marriage the one thing I can recall is there were never any arguments about money. She never concerned herself about it; as long as the bills were paid and we had "beach funds" she was okay. Oh, sure, she would question now and then if we could afford this or that, and I was always honest with her and frank in discussing the situation. As a matter of fact, most of the time she was never aware of how much money she had on her! On more than one occasion she called me to say we now owed this person or that person twenty bucks because they had decided to go out for lunch and she didn't have any money! After several of these little "loans," I began to hide "mad money" at different places in her wallet. She was very content with this idea, and when I checked her wallet on one occasion she had squirreled away quiet a bit of "mad money." I truly believe that, if a relationship is to last for a lifetime, this is one area where there can be no secrets and no lies. So many marriages fail because one partner or the other had, "money secrets".

In early 2003, retirement became a major topic of discussion, and after several months of negotiating with her that we would be financially secure, she decided to pursue the issue with her superiors. She would need what is known in government as an "early out retirement," meaning she had neither the time nor the age for normal retirement. There had never been an "early out" in her office. My employment retirement wasn't an issue. It had been determined by the administration where I worked that encouraging federal civil services employees to retire would be beneficial to the organization. So, on June 30, 2003, my wife officially retired at age fifty years and nine months, taking a small penalty for doing so. I soon followed, and August 28, 2003, was my last day working and my fifty-second birthday. I also took a penalty for retiring early.

We had put our Virginia home on the market in April after the decision to retire was finalized, expecting a quick sale. The quick sale did not happen, and as Mick's retirement time grew near she became very apprehensive about the decision, fearing the mortgage payment we would have to make on our retirement income. Her retirement day came and passed, my retirement day came and passed, and still no sale. By late November of 2003 we were both a little worried that we would have to retire in Virginia and pay the mortgage out of our retirement income, which would greatly affect our lifestyle in retirement, —plus, we were anxious to move to the beach and stay there full time. We needed the income the home sale would generate to build our new beach house. After seeing our home linger on the market for eight long months we were prepared to wait it out until springtime, but again, good things come to those that wait. We sold our home and the buyer wanted to wait until March of 2004 for settlement. This was a perfect scenario for us, as we did not want to start to build our retirement home in the wintertime.

After retirement and sale of our Virginia home we built another home for ourselves, this time with the intention this would be our last building adventure. My wife had recovered from her cancer issues and regular checkups had determined she was cancer free. This retirement home was built in the same location and on the very same lot where our beach house had stood since 1982. We thought about and even checked out the prospects of moving to Delaware, for tax reasons. But after extensive searches and finding that property as convenient as we were to the beach and other things was going to incur more expense we decided to stay right where we were, about two blocks from the beach on a quiet street with no through traffic. The one drawback to this scenario was the fact that we had to demolish the home we had learned to love for more than twenty years! As much as we hated that thought, we were preparing to do just that when a friend of a friend showed up at the door on his knees begging us not to tear it down. It seemed he had a vacant lot one street away, and he wanted to buy our house and move it. This was exactly the wish we had talked about; inasmuch as we had built the house ourselves some twenty years earlier and we had some emotional attachment to it. So the house was moved around the block, and we proceeded to build again, on the same lot as before, but twenty-one years later! Construction began in mid-April and continued for about six months, into November of 2004.

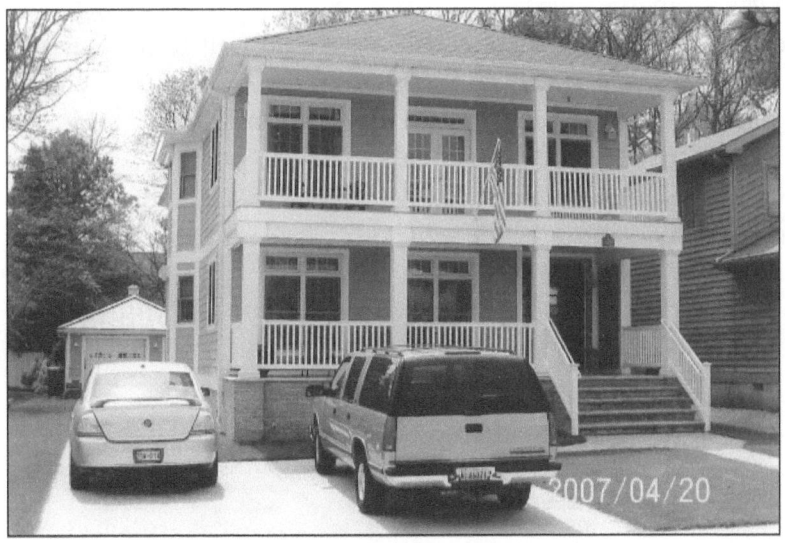

Our retirement home at the beach

We completed the new home and moved in Thanksgiving Day, 2004. It was a great and joyous time for her as she set about decorating it to fit her taste. I just stood back and let her go, for she had a special eye and talent for decorating. She used a combination of old and new, but our beach house retirement home was finally a place where she felt some of her special antique pieces belonged. She had collected many antique and unique pieces in our travels but somehow in the home we had just sold, she did not feel as if they "fit." This home she decorated in a kind of nautical theme, with all kinds of seashells, corals, prints, and real objects from the ocean. She had a special attachment to the beach, sea, and all things in it. There are fossils three million years old to shell mirrors that weigh at least three hundred pounds, mermaid paintings, plates with hand-painted shells, and things that could be just as well at home in a museum.

Even though we now lived at the beach and had been "weekend warriors" for many years, a few years ago she realized she couldn't take the sun anymore. I believe as we grew older the beach was not the attraction for us, it was the peace and serenity, away from the hustle and bustle where we could enjoy each other's company. On many days we would wait for the summer crowds to leave the beach in the afternoon so we could enjoy a quiet walk on the beach, watch the waves and the sea birds, and often watch as schools of dolphins would playfully swim by. I wrote the following poem for Mick in 1995 as she turned forty-three and began to see the value of a beach umbrella.

BEACHGOER

Her shoes are there, by the door
The magazines she read are on the floor
Her hat hangs on a nail in the wall
Her chair is leaning, about to fall.
She had returned from a trip to the shore
Just like a million times before
She needed to rest, so long in the sun
She remembers when suntans were fun.
In her younger years, recently passed
She disliked the clouds, the shadows they cast.
Now that she's on life's middle border,
Shadows and shade are a daily order.
She now loves the shells on the sand,
Especially the small ones, held in her hand.
In years gone by she paid them no mind,
Now each one's a treasure, a special find.
So, hat, shoes, magazine, and chair, they're all there
Sometimes to her life just isn't fair.
Because yesterday, she was young, so much meant so little
Now years are passing and she's in the middle.
So soon, maybe tomorrow, her stuff she'll gather,
Because it's at the shore she'd rather
Sit in the shade of umbrellas and clouds
To hear the ocean's tide, calling out loud.

But our joy was to be short-lived before devastating news, again.

On the Fourth of July weekend, 2005, we had a yard sale with neighbors to give other people our treasures. My wife mentioned all day she just felt "out of sorts." She described it as getting a little head rush as if one would stand suddenly, and said that she felt dizzy at times. The "C" word never entered our minds; we just thought she maybe had contacted a sinus infection or the problem might be something she had eaten. We didn't feel her symptoms were serious enough to warrant a doctor's visit, that is, not until July 12, 2005.

On this morning she came downstairs, and I noticed she was walking kind of leaning to her left and her color wasn't right; she was pale and stated she felt a little nauseous. I asked if she wanted to go to the emergency room and get checked out. First she said no, adding, "Just let me have some coffee and see how I feel." After about a half hour she changed her mind and said she thought it a good idea to go and get checked. We were still thinking, because of the issue with balance, that it was just a sinus infection or maybe an inner ear problem.

When we arrived at the emergency room the attending nurses and personnel did the usual stuff—blood pressure, temperature, pulse, etc. Then they put us into a room to await the doctor. The doctor came in, and the first thing was casual inquires about past health issues and such. He examined her neck and ears, checked the look of her sinus, and then—he took out his pencil from his pocket and asked her to follow it with her eyes, without turning her head. She followed the pencil, but even from my vantage point I could see her eyes darting back and forth. He immediately put away the pencil and said we should immediately have an MRI of her head.

The hospital staff came in momentarily, gave her a sheet to sign as consent for treatment, and explained the procedure that was about to happen. I waited in the emergency area while this was taking place, a thousand thoughts going through my mind. I think this was the first time I really thought about a brain tumor, not necessarily one from her breast cancer. After all, the doctors and all her prior medical discussions had always told us, and we had no reason to doubt, that after five years the likelihood of breast cancer returning was very slim. She had her regular checkups, as scheduled, and it had now been eight years and seven months since her first diagnosis. In addition to this she had been for her semiannual checkup just three months ago in April and had been given a clean slate. As a matter of fact, the actual doctor's note from that April checkup says, "Clinically no evidence of disease for eight years." So, reoccurrence of the disease was the last thing in my mind.

Shortly after the MRI of her head, we were waiting for the results in the ER and for some reason—I still never have gotten an explanation—but a nondenominational priest came and asked if we would like to pray. We both looked at each other and at the same time asked, "Is this bad news?" The priest looked kind of shocked, like we should have already been told something. He quickly recovered and mentioned that it was routine to pray with people in the ER. After praying and waiting about an hour, we were taken back to the original room. The original ER doctor came in and told us that the MRI was positive for a mass, and it was his and his colleague's position that in all probability it was "recurrent metastatic disease." He then explained that their suspicion was that the breast cancer had reoccurred in her right posterior cerebellar hemisphere in the form of a rather large tumor, which was behind her right ear right above the hairline. Further, the reason for her having nausea and balance issues was that the tumor was blocking drainage from this area of the brain, and the tumor, was having a mass effect on the forth ventricle. This tumor we were told was "extremely dangerous." It had an overall mass of 3.2 cm by 3.2 cm. This would covert in inches to about one and a quarter inches by one and a quarter inches, about the size of a walnut. This discovery is what reaffirms my belief that subsequent checkups after a diagnosis of positive lymph nodes should include annual scans of the entire body and brain.

The first treatment of any kind was a steroid called dexamethasone. This medication prevents fluid build-up and helps prevent swelling in the brain due to tumor pressure. It is much stronger than prednisone, and there were side effects that we did not like: sleeplessness, mental changes, increased appetite, and puffiness of her face. The increased appetite can be a good thing as many cancer patients lose appetite during treatment. Since she already had considerable pressure on her brain the doctor prescribed a dose of 12 mg per day and as symptoms warranted we had the option to increase or decrease the dosage.

Inasmuch as the doctor knew her history, he took it upon himself to contact a colleague in the radiation field and consult with him if it would be prudent to get a chest CT. With both doctors in agreement, we chose this scan also. While she was under going the chest CT I took the opportunity to contact the families and inform them the news was not good. Well, double whammy, the CT results were just as devastating with bad news! There was another walnut-sized tumor on her right paratracheal subcrarinal and right hilar adenopathy, and malignancy was suspected there. I know, you are asking, "Where and what is this?" This area is along the windpipe on the right side of the windpipe, mid-chest area and along with the hilar nodes area are actual lymph nodes in the chest area. Remember, lymph nodes are little "intersections" of blood vessels, and any cancer cells in any lymph node are likely to be carried in the bloodstream to other areas and organs of the body. This is called a metastasis and is always named for the original diagnosis, that is, breast cancer, colon cancer, etc. As it turns out, breast cancer that has became a metastasis in the brain is treated much differently than a cancerous tumor that originated in the brain.

As soon as we were able to bring our thoughts and emotions under control with a lot of tears and questions, we decided we should meet the radiation oncologist the ER doctor had consulted with and decide on a course of action. After consultation and answers to many questions it was decided by the medical experts that the clear and present danger was the brain tumor. Further is was decided among all involved that we should get a P.E.T. scan (Positron Emission Tomography), which uses a radioactive substance to produce a 3-D image of the body and associated organs, from the neck down. The P.E.T. scan is much more accurate than a CT. Over the course of her treatment and care for this disease, she would have nine of these scans! The first scan of this type, on July 15, 2005, was scary for both of us. First, the radioactive substance was delivered in a metal box, about the size of a shoebox, and it was marked with all kinds of hazard warnings and delivered by what looked like an armored truck!

During this first P.E.T. scan the procedure involved the injection with the radioactive substance, and a wait of about forty-five minutes for it to circulate through the bloodstream. I could not be in the same room during this procedure because of the radiation hazard. At this time the imaging machine would not allow for me to be in the room because of my pacemaker. This first machine actually moved the patient back and forth through a doughnutlike structure. Subsequently, after this first one, the new machine came into play. It moved back and forth, and the patient was allowed to lie still, and I was allowed to sit at the head of the machine and hold her hand, which was comforting to her because she was a little claustrophobic. When all was said and done, my wife would have this procedure nine times, along with twenty other scans, CTs, and MRIs, all in a period of two and a half years! I teased her that we could sit outside at night and tell which mosquitoes had bitten her because they would glow like fireflies!

Being scared and not very knowledgeable about issues relating to this or any type of brain surgery, we agreed to allow them to start the process by making an appointment with neurosurgeons in our area. This was done rather quickly, but not quick enough for us to go home, absorb what was happening, and say, "This is very serious, and we want to be sure we are getting the best possible doctors and results." After second thoughts we just could not picture brain surgery at our local hospital. One revealing thing that made us want to seek a more prominent facility was the literature given us about metastic brain tumors; it was to say the least, shocking. The statistics stated that there was only a 4 percent long-term survival rate, and patients usually succumb to the disease in four to eleven months after initial diagnosis. Fortunately for us, we had a neighbor down the street whose husband had a connection to the University of Maryland Medical Center in Baltimore. We really only knew them from the Ocean City neighborhood where we lived; they would pass and say hello, but we weren't really close as neighbors, yet. They were angels sent from heaven as they quickly became involved. The husband, within hours, had us an appointment with the head of the neurosurgery at this facility for July 14, 2005. We continued to use his expertise to answer questions about "doctor talk" for the next three years.

These two magnificent people were there with us at each Baltimore appointment and stayed close during the surgery and subsequent visits. As fate would have it, we had a connection to the doctor's wife that we never knew about—well, maybe not a connection, but a curious twist of fate. The doctor's wife had lost her only son in 1996; he had been in the navy stationed in North Island Naval Base on Coronado Island south of San Diego, California. My wife was on her work-related travel again, and I was traveling with her on this trip to North Island. On one particular morning I awoke, went for coffee and doughnuts, picked up a copy of a small paper called *Navy Times* or *Navy News*. The headline read, "Sailor found dead at sea." We did not know it then and we did not find out until sitting in the recovery room at UMMC on July 20, 2005, with our neighbors, that this sailor was her son. She and the doctor were in Germany at the time of his death, and we did not even know them at that time, but this was a curious twist of fate, which has lead to my having many conversations with her about the loss of a loved one and dealing with the heartache. She continues to this day to be someone I treasure because of this twist of fate and the great loss we have both had to deal with.

The consultation with the neurosurgeon, on July 14 went as we expected, although we were a bit surprised by his urgency to remove the brain tumor. It seems the urgency stems from the pressure on the left ventricle of the brain, which, within a short period, could cause seizures or death. He took the matter very seriously and actually moved another surgery, which was not nearly as urgent, so my wife could be scheduled. Her surgery appointment was July 20, 2005, at 9 a.m. The doctor's staff then took the ball and set up pre-op testing for Monday, July 18, 2005, at UMMC facilities.

The results of the P.E.T. were received back on July 18, 2005, and confirmed what the chest CT of July 13 had indicated—that there was in fact a mass in the right peritracheal and the right hilar node region, and the masses were consistent with metatastic disease. After the two doctors read these and consulted with us, we decided the chest issue could wait until the brain issue was resolved. It was thought by all involved that surgery to the brain with radiation afterward was the treatment of choice.

July 20, 2005, was anything but a typical day for us. We had come to Baltimore the night before and stayed a sleepless night in a hotel close to the UMMC, as the surgery was to start early, at 5:30 a.m. At this early time, we were to report to diagnostic imaging for another MRI of the brain and some computer guidance marking on my wife's scalp. It was during this check-in the first rather strange thing happened: upon check-in we were shocked to learn there were several other ladies in the medical center with the same first and last name as my wife! We quickly learned the importance of the ID bracelet and the equally important middle initial. As the technician began to shave little spots on her head we realized two more things: number one, these guys are not beauticians, and number two, she would probably be without her hair again soon. I stayed with her until she returned from the MRI. I offered positive thoughts and tried to keep her as positive as possible. I assured her, without being sure myself that she'd be ready to fuss with the doctors again in a few hours. From her past medical history, I knew she was always quick to recover, although we had never had any experience with anyone having brain surgery.

I was allowed to stay with her all during the preparations for the surgery, taking of vitals, and even until they started the anesthesia. As they wheeled her out into the hall and down the corridor of this massive facility she began to cry. When I asked her if she was okay, she said, "I love you and I hope I see you soon." At this point, the surgeon asked what seemed to me to be a strange question. He wanted to know if I had a cell phone. When I said I did, he proceeded to take down the number saying, "I'll call you when we get started and let you know how it is going." Mick and I were shocked that a surgeon would actually care enough to do this. I think it gave her some relief to know I would be made aware of the situation as the operation progressed. The surgeon did call about forty-five minutes into the operation to inform me he was "in" and he had not found anything he didn't expect to see. He said he would call me back when he had completed removal of the tumor. Another hour passed, and he called again to say his work was finished and the assistant would close up the incision. I would be able to see her in ICU in about a half hour. I took a deep sigh of relief and was anxious to see if she had all her faculties with her when the anesthetic was gone.

As family, friends, and I waited in the ICU waiting area, we spoke of how she had influenced us all. Everyone could see the influence she had on my life; she was more than half the reason we were at the place we were in our lives, and she was the inspiration for many things I had written over the years. It was her willingness to go along with my crazy building-our-own-home ideas. One friend that had been our partner for many years in the Ocean City beach house recalled how she had convinced him to use her method to get rid of his hiccupping episode. She apparently had told him to put a paper bag over his head and breathe into it; this, she said, would end his hiccups. Well, after about a half hour of watching the bag expand and contract, she was so hysterical with laughter she was in tears.

One of my brothers remembered how she was at Christmas, always laughing and full of mischief. She had many years earlier started a tradition of giving gag gifts to various members of my family. Once this tradition was started we carried it on for many years. Family members would search all year for the perfect inexpensive gag gift to surprise the entire family with. I remember she gave my baby sister a tricycle. You see, my little sister is very small, and she had been selling raffle tickets at a local race track on Saturday night, walking for miles, so this gag gift was for her to "cruise the pits" selling raffle tickets from her tricycle. My younger brother had affection for dinosaurs, so for many years his gag gift was—you guessed it—a dinosaur of some sort. She also bought as gag gifts Fisher-Price toy tool sets for my brothers that were into home remodeling, toy trucks for the brother into trucking, toy phone for the niece who you could not get off the phone, and many, many more gifts that gave us many memories of laughter at Christmas. She will be missed, and Christmases will be quiet without her around.

Sure enough, just as the doctor had said, the orderlies came wheeling her down the hall. To my surprise she was sitting up smiling, and she waved to me. There was a friend with me whom she had not seen in a few years; she immediately recognized him and called him by his name! She was back and had all her faculties, and within an hour she was asking for something to eat! She spent the next two days having some minor therapy to assure all that her sense of balance and walking ability had not been impaired. And to our amazement she was well enough to be discharged forty-eight hours after major brain surgery. We then asked to stay an extra night because we lived about a hundred and sixty miles from the UMMC campus. Should a problem occur it would be difficult to get her back to that facility with any haste. The doctors agreed to our request for another night's stay, and my wife was discharged on July 23, 2005, with a follow-up appointment on July 27.

July 27 was a busy day for us as we had two or three doctors to see, and we had to decide a course of action. The first doctor was the neurosurgeon for the follow-up. We were excited to learn he felt he had "excised 99.9 percent of this tumor" and that the staples could be removed next week. An appointment was scheduled for the following Wednesday, August 3, 2005, to do just that. After this first appointment there were two more doctors on the agenda for that day, the breast cancer doctor and a radiation oncologist.

August 3 arrived after another sleepless night with my wife worrying about the pain that was going to be inflicted with removal of the staples from her head. As it would turn out, her fears were complete unfounded. The removal of the staples took less than five minutes, and she did not even realize they had been removed. She thought the nurse was just preparing the area to remove them when in fact she was pulling them out! After the staples were removed we could see there was going to be about a three-inch scar up the back of her head about an inch right of center, and in all likelihood, hair would never grow in this area. A small price to pay for what had been a deadly situation. The most dangerous of the tumors was excised, and now we could move on to the situation "below the neck."

Upon discharge the neurosurgeon's staff had, at our request, set up a consultation with a world-renowned breast cancer oncologist. She practiced there at the UMMC, and we could see her when we returned for the post-op checkup of Mick's head. The first decision did not relate to a health issue; as I mentioned before, these guys are surgeons, not beauticians. The site of the surgery was shaved to the skin but only in about a three-inch wide swath up the back of her head, with twenty-one staples that looked like a railroad track. So, here come the old clippers from 1997, and I get to practice my marine haircut style again. This time it wasn't as emotional as back in 1997, but it was still sad because she had grown her hair back long enough to have a ponytail again. We sat on the back porch of our home and proceeded to cut all the remaining hair from her head; I don't know why, but this time I saved a large clump in an envelope. Maybe secretly in my mind I knew she would never have hair again.

The next decision that we faced was much more important, deciding upon a treatment for the issue with the paratracheal region of her chest. This involved a whole new set of doctors and procedures and, as with any cancer issue, it seems that there is a specialist for each of the different areas where it occurs. We had an appointment set up for July 27, 2005, at UMMC, the same day we were to return for the follow-up appointment with the neurosurgeon, with a world-renowned breast cancer specialist and research doctor. This specialist is kind of a GP of all breast cancers and specializes in metastasis cancer.

Well, it turns out that there are several options to treat reoccurring mestastic breast cancer and a lot depended on the pathological report of the tumor removed from Mick's brain. The tumor had been sent to the lab, and results proved the tumor was consistent with a "a primary lesion in the breast." meaning it was, in fact, all doubt removed, a metastatic reoccurrence of beast cancer from the 1996 issue. It was apparent that the nasty cancer cells had fallen asleep for a while and had now decided to wreak havoc again. The choice of drug to prescribe for treatment would hinge on whether the tumor was *ER positive or negative,* (estrogen receptor positive or negative). If the tumor were positive, that would mean it depends on estrogen to grow; of course, a negative finding would mean it gets its growing capability from other sources. Treatments for ER negative cancers are much more limited.

Another important test on the cancer is to determine if the cells are HER2 negative or positive. What is this? Well, the long name is *Human Epidermal growth factor Receptor 2.* A test kind of gives an indication as to how aggressive the cancer uses a protein to grow. The answer will dictate a cancer treatment drug to combat the disease. It seems that about 25 percent of breast cancers are HER2 positive, meaning the cells are able to grow like weeds in a garden! They have these little messengers that talk to each other through the cell walls and can divide and become more cancer cells quickly. It should be noted that good cells have these receptors, too, and it is a protein also necessary for good cell growth.

The pathological test results from the lab indicated our tumor was *ER-positive,* meaning the cancer cells were dependent on estrogen to grow, so—common sense would tell you that—reducing the estrogen or eliminating it would help in the fight against this cancer. There were at the time several new medicines on the market to do this, one of which is in a group of medicines called letrozoles. These medicines are used for treatment of advanced breast cancers, usually stage three and four. After considering our options we chose a letrozole by the trade name of Femara. The prescribed dosage depends on every situation being different, and the goal is to reduce the amount of estrogen available for the little cancer cell suckers to eat, so some of them starve. The second test of the cancer cells from our tumor gave a little bit more encouraging news as the results of the HER2 test revealed the cells were in fact HER2/NEU, meaning the cancer was not real aggressive. Aggressive is kind of a relative term when used by doctors versus a patient. What is termed "not aggressive" to the doctors sometimes means panic in a patient, especially when things seem to change weekly.

So, after all this, what am I saying? I want to pass on the need for having the tumor tested or a biopsy done to find out about the previously mentioned tests. The tests indicate a treatment protocol or a medicine that will have the best result for one who is given diagnosis of reoccurring breast cancer.

At this time I want to tell the story of another type of test that helps your oncologist kind of track cell growth. This blood test is commonly referred to as a "tumor marker test." A tumor marker is a substance found in blood; when found at elevated levels, it can indicate cancer growth. The medical establishment has determined, by some means, that a level, for a nonsmoker, should less than 2.5ng/ml. I, not being a doctor, have a problem with this test being used after one has cancer as a tool to detect cancer growth. I would think one would need to know a baseline reading, prior to any cancer, and then read the levels periodically. If there is a rise in the reading, then take a serious look for cancer. My skepticism of this test and its reliability stems from our experience with the readings derived, and our subsequent letdowns from them. I will detail this later in my cancer story.

Also on this day, July 27, we consulted with radiation doctors about something called "full brain radiation." It seems the renowned breast cancer specialist is not a big fan of this treatment, although she did defer our questions to the specialist. It now appears, with the ability to use hindsight, that the specialist downplayed the side effects, mentioning only maybe a "ringing in the ears and some dry eyes." We had already done a little research on our own and knew there were actually several more serious side effects that were possible. In addition to "ringing in the ears," you can suffer hearing loss, serious memory problems, headaches, speech problems, eye problems, and, in rare cases, even fatal side effects. The radiation specialist also gave us some odds of tumors returning to the brain with and without radiation therapy. According to him, after radiation therapy the odds of a tumor returning anywhere in the brain were about fifty-fifty, with only a 10 percent chance of a reoccurrence at the original site. Without the radiation therapy, the odds increased to a 70 percent chance of return somewhere in the brain and a greater than 20 percent chance a tumor would regrow at the original site. After learning these odds we wanted to take the best shot we had at never having to deal with brain tumors again, so we decided to go for the full brain therapy. During this consultation we learned that, even though radiation is a specialized field, as long as a facility has the most modern equipment treatment, regimens are basic stuff. We were pleased to hear this, as it would enable us to get the radiation treatment close to home.

Tuesday, August 2, 2005, was the day for actual set-up for the radiation therapy. The set-up involved the making of a plastic mask, form fitted to Mick's face, which would be bolted to the table of the radiation machine to assure her head was held in the same location during each treatment. This mask kind of resembles a plastic hockey mask; the technician heats up the plastic, then pushes it over the patient's face to conform to the nose, eyes, and chin. My wife said this was a very scary experience. She asked the technician to cut through the plastic around her eyes and nose. After this initial mask-making ceremony, the first of fifteen radiation treatments to her brain was set to begin on August 9, 2005. The actual treatment time for each appointment was only about forty-five seconds, but my wife hated the almost five minutes she had to be behind that mask bolted to a table! She chose to have her treatment early in the day so she could have the rest of the day to do "normal things," carrying on with her vow from 1996 to be "as normal as possible."

By the end of August 2005, the radiation had ended, and I could see her at times sitting around just kind of staring into space, thoughts deep in her illness. I asked her if she thought it would help if she had something to occupy her mind and keep her a little busy, kind of engage her mind with something outside of treatments and cancer. She admitted it was becoming more and more difficult to be normal as possible and perhaps some responsibility would be good therapy. Since she thought it might be a good idea, I made contact with her former boss and asked for his help. He had always been very close to us, kind of like another brother. Within a matter of days he had arranged for her to do some administrative work through a contractor. Her hours were flexible; she could work whenever she wanted and for as long as she wanted. This turned out to be a great part of her recovery. She would work about twenty-seven hours a month, but I think just the feeling of being useful kept her spirits up.

She realized she could contribute and be functional even though she was in the fight of her life. She joyfully set about doing the things assigned her and even enjoyed the visits back to her old office. She continued to do this small job right up until a couple of weeks before her end.

During this start to our recovery and treatment we found out that a bone scan was in order to check for problems with her bones. The main question was, had the cancer spread to these areas? The bone scan involves injecting some foreign substance that I'm convinced probably shouldn't be in our bodies.

Also, it was decided that she should continue taking the steroid pill because the radiation treatment can cause some swelling in the brain. This was not good news to my wife as she had learned to despise this medicine because of her inability to sleep, and fat face. As treatment and the disease progressed the need for steroids became more and more evident.

Well, the results proved to be negative for cancer but ironically, she now had a sinus infection—what we had originally thought to be the source of her lightheadedness and feeling funny back in July before the tumor discovery. The bone scan showed a serious infection, and at first we thought the doctors would treat it with antibiotics. But, after much consideration, they decided to let the infection alone until the end of radiation since there appeared to be no pain or discomfort associated with it. As it turned out, a subsequent bone scan proved the infection went away on its own.

Remember the Femara medicine prescribed for the treatment of the rest of the cancer located in her chest area?

Well, she took the first pill on August 7, 2005, and this would continue to be a daily routine, along with a steroid pill for several weeks. The steroids would end, temporarily, but the Femara would continue until it seems to lose its ability to fight the disease. Although Femara has several possible side effects, my wife only experienced a couple and they were mild; she had an increase in hot flashes and some bone pain, especially in her legs.

As time went along and the radiation treatments continued I recalled that during our first battle in 1997 I had made meals that were high in protein to keep up her energy level. Again I began my daily cooking to try and increase her intake of protein, using fresh fish supplied by a neighbor, fresh greens and chicken, turkey, and also an increase in red meat. This had worked well then to combat the dying protein cells killed off by the radiation. I think from a firsthand experience, this diet helped, and we were able to keep her somewhat close to normal.

Beginning about the end of the radiation treatments Mick was beginning to feel fatigued a lot more. She really had to push herself to continue her daily walks and exercise. I, being the eternal optimist, tried to keep her upbeat, even though I don't know that I could be as strong as she was through this ordeal. It is always just as easy to think, say and do something positive, as it is to think, do, or say something negative. As I wrote in my diary on September 25, 2005:

> *"Today, September 25, starts out a bad day, Bren is tired and uninspired, I have to work really hard to get her out of bed and to stop just lying on the couch. Hopefully we will exercise today, walking for a while, it helps her, me, because when she is active it gives me hope. After all, when she feels bad or has an off day, so do I. I lose my mate, my partner, and my best friend. This illness I realize will take some time to control, but control is what we pray for".*

Her moods seemed to go up and down day by day, from feeling good and resilient, to being very fatigued. This feeling of fatigue was mostly due to the radiation effects; after all, we were told it could take as long as six months for the radiation to work its way out. Meanwhile, the medication Femara continued. Taking this medicine required monthly checkups, blood work, and a trip to Baltimore to do this each time. It also required more scans to check on the chest region to see if the medicine was truly having an effect. The first such scan was a CT of the chest on October 21, which indicated that there was a "slight decrease in the size of a few right hilar lymph nodes." I must say at this point, it is very important to be sure the facility one chooses to have perform these scans has access to all scans. This is because in order to track size and growth of tumors or lesions they must have something to compare. We started, from the very first scans from the emergency in July of 2005 up until the very last one in July of 2008, to carry copies of these with us. Technology has advanced enough that the scans are now downloaded to a disk.

On many of our trips to and from Baltimore she would always insist on a little diversion to antique hunt or a mall-shopping trip. I think these stops along the way to treatment were another way she felt she was living "as normal as possible," and they gave her diversion from the very serious issue at hand.

Scans, scans, and more scans! There were to be two more scans in 2005, both in December. The first was a nuclear medicine PET that gave us a little uplift as this scan showed no increase and no new activity regarding cancer. This result was backed up a few days later with a simpler CT scan.

After the two scans of December 2005, we decided for the first time in our married life we would not be home or see some of our family at Christmas. Instead, we would go to Florida—sunshine and palm trees for Christmas! This Christmas was very unusual, in a good kind of way, for us both. We got to enjoy the warmth and comfort of my brother's home, and there was something Mick had been longing to see at a show in Miami—the King Tut exhibit. I was surprised that she wanted to see this because she was never the museum type. She kind of felt like, "Hey, if you can't touch it or buy it, what's the point?" We, having lived in the northern Virginia area, were very close to many museums, but she had visited very few. But this exhibit

R. Lee Hall

she had been interested in for years, and she had tracked its show places and dates closely. So on Christmas Day we drove from the west coast of Florida to Miami to see this extraordinary exhibit, and even though it was much more crowded than we imagined, she enjoyed this immensely. She talked about it with fascination and was able to put aside her health issues for that day.

In late March of 2006—yep, we finally got to 2006—the radiation doctor wanted to do an MRI of her brain to check for anything new there. This test gave us even more good feelings because once again, "no new lesions identified." Another month went by, and two more scans were ordered: a chest CT, without "contrast." What is contrast? You are wondering. Well, contrast is when they actually inject a substance, much like a dye, into the bloodstream. This substance will produce a clearer picture as irregularities are highlighted. In my opinion, though I'm not a doctor, when scans are necessary, I would think it prudent to want as clear picture as possible. The scans are done with and without contrast. Also in late April a CT of her pelvis was done, this one with contrast, and a nuclear medicine CT whole body scan of the bones. To our joy these scans showed no increases or new suspect sites for cancer; the results from both stated "no definite evidence of new metastatic disease."

By mid-2006 we had been on the Femara regimen for almost ten months with no new activity present. Remember that I talked about the blood work and a reading called a "tumor marker?" These readings were a regular thing each time we visited the doctors in Baltimore, and all indications were that the Femara was working, as the numbers steadily decreased.

During the time between November of 2005 and early 2006 we had good feelings that we were beating the disease, or at least holding our own against it. We didn't let anything hold us back. We continued to live our life as normally as possible. We traveled to Florida to help relatives remodel a house; we traveled to Vegas for a delayed anniversary trip I had planned—she had wanted to see Celine Dion, but because of the 2005 reoccurrence and surgery it did not happen in 2005. We went to Massachusetts for flea markets. Mick never complained about the disease, nor did it appear to have slowed her down much! She was pretty much the picture of health, and even though she had the issue with the tumor in her chest, the doctors kept remarking that the only way you could tell she had cancer was to look at a picture! She was still walking a couple of miles each day, riding her bike, doing her part-time consulting job, and doing many things associated with the remodeling of our relatives' Florida home. She was especially fond of the demolition parts! She nearly wore my sister-in-law out traveling the roads to flea markets, shops, antique shows, and such. Looking back now, I realize that she always seemed to be in a hurry. Maybe she had been given a sign to live quickly, for time was getting short.

In early May of 2006 we decided that, inasmuch as her cancer had became a monitoring situation, we would like to be closer to home for the checkups. We asked the Baltimore doctors for a reference to someone closer to our home. As it turns out, the doctor they recommended wasn't to our liking. Upon our initial meeting and consultation, we got an uneasy feeling about the doctor. The first thing was that she read my wife's medical history and looked shocked. We got the feeling she was thinking, "My goodness, how is this lady still alive and looking this well?" After that she immediately ordered another bone scan of the spine; we had just had two done! This doctor also, to us, had an attitude like, "Your cancer is going to kill you, so I'll just make the motions, collect my fee until this cancer thing ends." This particular doctor made us so uneasy we decided to try other doctors even closer to our home.

As it would turn out, this was a wise decision because if you feel uneasy about the treatment you are getting and unsure the doctor is going to try his or her best, it will have a negative effect on the treatment process overall. I think that during the course of treatment for any illness, you should not have a fear of changing doctors. You can take all records with you, and one thing we must remember is that the doctors work for us. We went to the radiation oncologist we were seeing and asked for him to recommend someone he would trust with his wife and family. He recommended a local doctor with extensive experience in all types of cancer. Upon first meeting my wife felt that he really cared for his patients. What's more, he agreed to let us keep the Baltimore doctors in the loop; as a matter of fact, he would later have conversation and correspondence with them. So, with the situation being as it was, a kind of a monitoring treatment with regular blood work and exams, we switched to a doctor seventeen miles from our home with the condition we return to Baltimore every six months or as need arose.

On August 4, 2006, we began treatment under the local doctor's care. He agreed with the treatment program so far but wanted Mick to get a regular mammogram since it had been a couple of years since she had last gone through one. With bated breath we had this done, and, again, good news; the mammogram was normal. Her mammograms had always been normal going all the way back to 1995, the year she began to have them.

On the morning of September 14, 2006, my wife began to have issues with her eyes. In her words, "They seem to be moving in slow motion." I tried moving a pencil in front of her eye, much like the original emergency room doctor had done about a year earlier. It was then I noticed, sure enough, her left eye when coming back from movement to the left was very slow, kind of like a lazy eye. We make an appointment with the radiation doctor because we knew that one side effect could be eye and vision problems. The doctor explained to us there could be some muscle and nerve damage done by the radiation, which would cause such a problem, but as a precaution he wanted another—MRI of the brain. The MRI proved to be good news, no abnormalities detected! We decided to seek an eye specialist. He seemed to think the problems were nerve related. To compensate, perhaps stronger reading glasses were in order, but he made no determination as to the reason for the vision problems.

This eye problem would become more persistent and bothersome to her over the course of the next few months. Now, with the invaluable knowledge of Mr. Hindsight, I think this was the beginning of more tumors in her brain. Even though the MRI of September 27, 2006, had shown no abnormalities, I am inclined to believe the beginning of what was to be deadly was actually starting now, and perhaps the MRI somehow missed detecting it.

As I have written before, there was blood work done each appointment we had. Mick's arm got stuck so much they finally had to stick her in the hand just to get any samples! We had been on the Femara since August of 2005, and now we were approaching 2007. We had blood work done, and the results for the tumor marker test indicated a rise in this reading, which would indicate there could be increased activity relating to cancer cells. So—another scan, this time another PET, the one with the nuclear stuff.

The results are alarming, but not devastating. The scan showed that there actually was increased size in the chest lymph node area. The doctor reading the scan had failed to compare it with the most recent PET. He had gone back to the scan done on December of 2005 and missed the newer one from April of 2006. We brought this to his attention and he did another comparison. When he compared these two, lo and behold, we got bad news! This scan appeared to show that the liver was now getting involved as there seemed to be a small growth on the right lobe. Well, after consultation with the doctors, both local and in Baltimore, it seemed the little cancer cell dudes had found a way to get around the Femara medicine and now had a new diet of something other than estrogen.

Inasmuch as it seemed the Femara had run its course, the doctors thought we should explore another question as well. Regarding the chest area, they wanted to know if it was really breast cancer. The thought was that an ENT doctor might be able to obtain a biopsy by going down the throat and extracting a sample, just to be sure we weren't dealing with another cancer such as lung cancer. If the test proved it to be lung cancer, then another whole set of rules and medicines would apply. Well, after much to-do and miscommunication between doctors, and frustration on our part, we decided to take a step back, catch our breath, and head to Florida, putting any treatment, exams, or new medicines on hold until we returned. We left for Florida on February 23, 2007.

On this Florida trip there would be more remodeling with demolition involved— remember, Mick is the demo gal! In the circular drive of my brother's home the previous homeowner had constructed this monstrosity he called a fountain. My brother and sister-in-law hated it. Mick decided that, while we did other jobs, landscaping, tree trimming and such, she would demo the fountain. Remember, this is a lady currently on cancer therapy and less than a year and a half removed from major brain surgery! Well, she proceeded over the next four days to beat and pound the old blocks, tile, and concrete into submission and all that was left was a hunk of concrete about a foot thick and about four feet square. My brother and I were using a bucket truck to trim trees and I had a good observation point. I could see she was getting nowhere, getting frustrated and sweating like a pig. I looked at my brother and said, "We're going to have help dragging palm limbs in a minute." Sure enough, she strolled up to our pile and began dragging the palm limbs to the street. I asked her what the problem was with the concrete and she replied, "It's harder than your head, come help me." I did go to her aid; I held the chisel while she struck it with a twelve-pound sledge. Looking back now, I must have been crazy—after all she was having eye problems. But I trusted her to hit the chisel and not me. Not only did she hit it, but the chisel eventually gave out, bending so much we could no longer use it. I think she was proud of what she had accomplished. Indeed, it made her feel "as normal as possible."

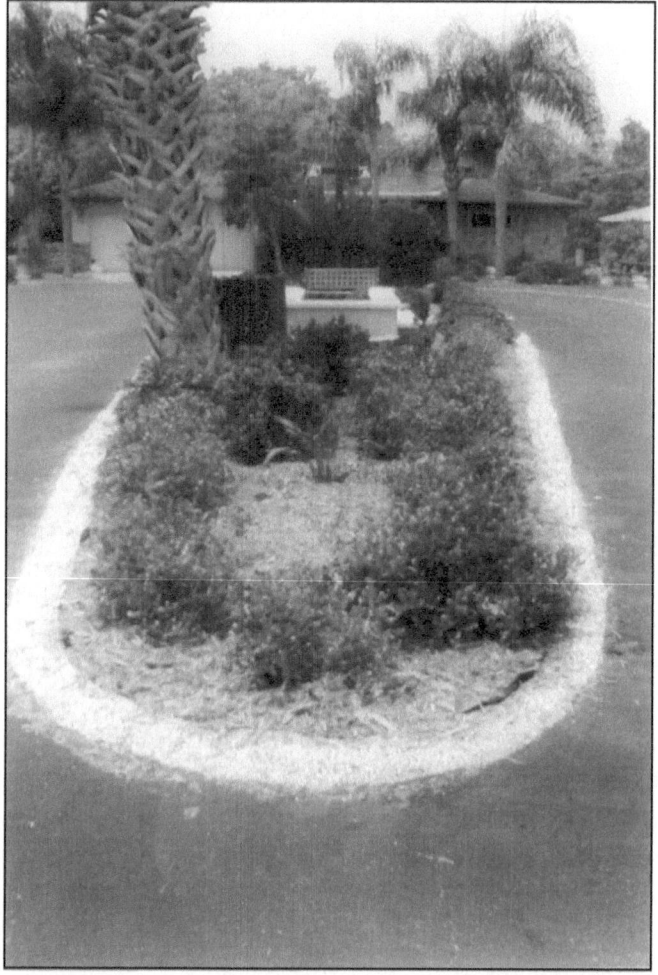

The circular drive in Florida, with the old fountain

Finally, on March 23, 2007, the biopsy of the paratracheal region was done, and preliminary test proved it is in fact breast cancer, although the lab would have liked more sample to test, being there was about a 5 percent chance they were lung cancer cells. The only way a bigger sample could be obtained was surgery through the throat—not an option in our minds. We were content in our belief and the odds being 95 percent that these were breast cancer cells. We decided to stay the course and get new ammunition to fight the cancer.

Not so fast. The doctors decided to continue with the Femara for a couple of months, then recheck the tumor markers, do another PET, and go from there. The next nuclear injection for the PET was scheduled for May 21, 2007. This test revealed more disappointing news, the biggest of which was that the small spots on the liver had now increased to two tumors, one of 24 mm and one of 14 mm, confirming increasing hepatic (liver) metastatic disease. The doctor near our home wanted us to go back to our doctor in Baltimore for more input as to where we should be heading. And he was surprised once again that Mick was having "no adverse effects from the disease." We asked about possible surgery to the liver to remove these newfound problem spots. Our question was met with a definitive "not a good idea," since the surgery is invasive and might in the short term decrease her quality of life. Further research has shown that removal of metastic tumors of the liver doesn't provide any life extension over treatment with drugs. There is also a process called chemoembolization, which delivers a large dose of a chemo medicine directly into the liver tumor. This treatment depends largely upon whether the tumor is "in" or "on" the liver, because often location tells the story of where the tumor gets its blood supply.

After weighing all options, the new cancer weapon of choice was a drug called Xeloda, pronounced with the X sounding like a Z. The generic name for this drug is capecitabine. This drug was one of the first chemotherapy drugs which can be taken orally. It is usually taken in fourteen-day cycles with seven days off between cycles, and is often given in large dosage, as many as fourteen pills a day, taken twice a day. Our doctors were in agreement with us to start with a medium dosage and gauge the results. This meant Mick would be taking seven pills a day, four in the morning and three in the afternoon. One of the dreaded side effects of this medicine is the hand/foot syndrome. This side effect causes the hands and feet to dry and crack and become very sore. My wife suffered this side effect, not so much on the hands, but her feet were cracked and dry through the entire time on this medicine. There are other side effects, but she was fortunate not have to deal with those; again, she tolerated another chemo drug with the fortitude of a champion! There was another drug, very new to breast cancer treatment, which we considered using even though it was designed for use in colon cancers. Its name was abraxane. Where do they come up with these names? This is an intravenous drug given in a doctor's office, and there are side effects that need to be addressed before anyone should consider this drug. Again, I'm not a doctor, and I would urge anyone faced with decisions to weigh all their options and use doctors you are comfortable with, and be active in any decision making! As it turned out, this drug became less of an option for us because of the previous history of a brain tumor. It seems this medicine could induce bleeding in the brain.

So our new ammo was the drug Xeloda, a dose of 3500 mg a day, seven pills taken four in the morning and three in the afternoon. My wife liked the convenience of pill versus anything that had to be injected. Even though I had been her pill record-keeper for the past year and a half, I now had taken to writing each and every dose down, because so much was being given that I found it difficult to remember it all. But, looking back now, I think perhaps the Xeloda along with an injected chemo would have proven to be more of a weapon. We had given some thought to using an adjuvant drug along with this one. But I can't dwell on what might have been. We made our choice after seeking the best advice and consultation we thought available, and we were willing to stand by our decision. We always felt, and never changed our conviction, that Mick should not take any treatment that could be worse than the disease. She would often say, "What good would it be to know you are defeating the cancer, but becoming a vegetable?" She opted for quality of life and remained true to her commitment to be "as normal as possible."

As normal as possible included another trip to Florida without relatives so we could get away from doctors and medicine. We decided to go during an off cycle from the Xeloda. This meant she had seven days of freedom from anything! There was more demolition to be done in the Florida house. First, there was this hideous concrete wall-looking thing as you entered from the garage. It was supposed to look like rocks. My brother and his wife had given us permission to demolish this thing. Well, we thought it was fake rocks but *noooo*—it was actual concrete sculpted to look like rock. My wife whaled on it with a small hammer to no avail, then looked at me and said, "I'm gonna need a bigger hammer." We bought one, and she proceeded over the next few days pounding the wall into submission. An amazing accomplishment considering she was in the fight of her life, but this was what she considered to be as normal as possible. We spent a wonderful couple of weeks running around southern Florida, collecting her favorite things—shells, antiques, and sharks' teeth—in addition to doing more remodeling to the Florida house. She was the type who would not allow any of us to sit still during daytime hours. She was a little slow in the mornings, but once she got you going, there was no stopping her till dark!

In early July of 2007 the issue with her eyes was becoming more pronounced. She complained that she was seeing double at times and trying to focus was becoming a problem. Again we went to see the radiation doctor and mentioned this to our oncology doctor. They both were inclined to believe this was an effect from the full brain radiation and recommended we see an eye specialist. We made an appointment to have her eyes and vision checked. After we arrived at the eye clinic, met the doctor, and gave a history of our situation, he began his exam. It was at this time I saw, by looking over his shoulder, the strange behavior she had been describing about her vision. When the doctor passed a light by her eye, her left eye would follow the beam to the right, but then it very slowly would return to center, a kind of delayed reaction. His diagnosis was something called esotropia, or sixth nerve palsy. He was of the opinion this was residual effect of the radiation, and there wasn't a cure. It might get better with time as the radiation continued to dissipate; however, he could provide some relief by providing a special set of glasses that would redirect the light into her left eye.

Having little choice but to have the glasses made and hope for correction, we had our doubts about improvement. After all, it had now been almost two years since the full brain radiation. Again, here I want to interject the wisdom of old Mr. Hindsight. I now suspect strongly that the eye problem was in all likelihood the beginning of tumor growth in the left front of her brain, or perhaps even the start of the tumor on the brain stem. But we failed, the doctors failed, to connect the dots and request another MRI of her brain at this time. Would it have made a difference? Who knows? Her eye problems continued and worsened all the way to the end.

By September 27, 2007, we had been on the Xeloda cycles since May and everyone agreed that blood work tumor marker readings were beginning to decrease substantially. The doctors thought this would be a good time for—are you ready?—another nuclear PET scan! We had high hopes that the blood work was an indication the disease was under control. Our hopes were upheld, and we were elated to find "interval improvement of the metastatic disease when compared to the 5/21/07 scan." In fact, for the first time since the onset of this ordeal, the lymph nodes in the chest area are smaller and demonstrate "decreased hypermetabolic activity." And to top it off, the hepatic (liver) lesions appeared to be smaller and one of them had decreased activity. The icing on the cake—"no new abnormalities identified."

This scan gave us a great deal of hope that we were finally turning a corner on this nasty disease and perhaps we had found our "miracle drug." Other than the complaints about her eyes, my wife felt good, and there were no visible signs of cancer on the outside. Again, doctors remarked that you would never know she had cancer unless you looked at a picture, and this picture even seemed to show a brighter outlook. We decided we could live with the side effects of the Xeloda. The skin rash and hand/foot syndrome were the most bothersome.

The decision was to continue the Xeloda, but reduce it to 3000 mg a day—oh, boy!—one less pill. She had been taking seven, and now it would only be six. The cycle would continue to be fourteen days with pills, seven days without, then blood work after each cycle. I kept track of her medicines religiously, and she'd always ask, "Which one is this, and why am I taking it?" The first full brain radiation had left her short-term memory somewhat sparse.

Her memory wasn't always deficient. I can remember one of trips to the flea market in Brimfield, Massachusetts. My sister had accompanied us, and she had purchased an old print of a bird looking at his reflection in a fountain. Upon seeing the print my wife immediately said, "I know where the original is for that." I thought to myself, *now how can she remember that in all the thousand of vendors here at Brimfield?* Well, it turns out the original wasn't even at Brimfield. She said she had seen it years before at a shop in Delaware. I doubted her accuracy and thought surely it must have been a similar painting. But upon our return to the Delaware area, we revisited the shop where she claimed the "original" was, and, lo and behold, her memory had not failed her nor had it played tricks on her. In fact, we purchased the original, had it restored, and gave it to my sister for Christmas. It turns out the artist actually has some paintings in the National Gallery of Art, but the strange thing is that even after the full brain radiation she still had an uncanny ability to remember where all the antique shops were between New England and Florida!

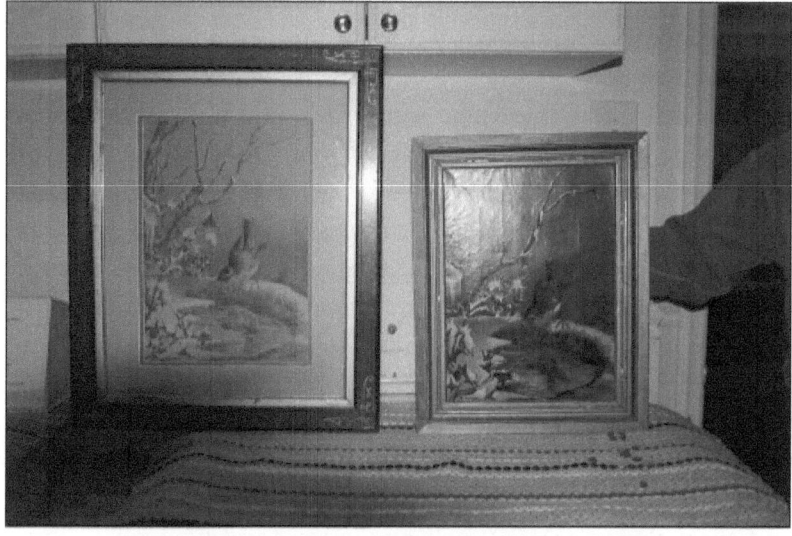

The print is on left and the original on the right; her memory served her well

Remember back in the chapter called "Recovery and Moving" on relating to the 1997 cancer issue? Well, that same cousin now had battled for nine years, and her prognosis was not at all encouraging news to my wife and I. It seems she had now developed brain tumors and lesions and had now had medical treatment that would have a direct impact on future decisions we made. This was heartbreaking, to say the least, because this cousin had used Xeloda along with other medicines we were investigating. The last time we saw her was in May 2007. She was also cut from the same mold as my wife: independent, strong, and never letting the disease get her down. But by November she had radiation surgery on lesions on her brain. This surgery left her unable to swallow, unable to speak above a whisper, and without the ability to close her right eye or straighten out her legs.

It appears she chose to let her radiation oncologist do stereotatic surgery on six lesions at one time. From all the information we were able to gather, this is really aggressive. The usual treatment of this type is three tumors or lesions at a time, never six. Did her doctors get a little too aggressive with the treatment? When we paid her a visit in November, we were left stunned by her condition. It left a big impact on our future decision-making and the path we chose.

We continued on the Xeloda through October, November, and into mid-December with each tumor marker reading from the blood work decreasing. It had, by mid-December, decreased from a reading of 27.1 in August of 2005 to an all time low of 3.9 on December 19, 2007. (Remember, 2.5 is a normal reading.)

This was such good news that our doctors agreed we could probably stop the Xeloda because we didn't want to take the chance of the same thing happening as with the Femara, that being that the little cancer suckers found another road to travel and became immune to the medicine. But in order to get a confirmation of our good news another—you guessed it—PET scan! But it could wait till early January as we were—you guessed it again— going back to Florida! Remember, this is the lady that all through out this ordeal wanted to be as normal as possible, and I guess in her mind these were the things she would be in fact be doing if everything was "normal."

While we were in Florida, on January 9, 2008, sad news came to us. Mick's cousin with the breast cancer had lost her battle and passed. She was still going until the end. Although she had been in a half vegetative state for about two months, her son had taken her to California chasing a treatment that they had hoped she could tolerate and extend her life with quality. This was an extremely hard bit of news to take, as this cousin was one year younger than my wife, and there were uncanny similarities in the progression of the disease in each case.

After a winter break to Florida, in which Mick actually increased her walks and exercise, she was so happy about the CEA readings and their decrease she seemed to push herself to be as normal as possible. We came back to a scheduled PET/CT scan to be done on January 15, 2008. This scan even began a little differently from those in the past, as the waiting time after injection of the nuclear contrast agent had now been increased from sixty minutes to ninety minutes in order to give the nuclear stuff more time to settle in. The results were given on January 16—devastating news and dashed hopes!

The scan of disappoint began with the first statement. "There is drastic progression of metastatic disease." (Remember, a PET is a scan from the neck down; it doesn't include the head or brain.) There was—ready for this?—a lesion on the T-9 vertebral body; a new bony mestastasis on the lateral right midrib; worsening activity in the pretracheal and hilar lymph nodes; new hypermetabolic activity in the subcarinal region (the esophagus near the lung); multiple areas scattered throughout the liver; a new area of activity in the left adrenal gland; and new activity in the left and right ileum, which are the bones of the pelvis. All the readings were substantiated by the CT part of this scan, as if news this bad needed backup!

We now knew that the CEA tumor marker reading had given us false hope, and from this point on, I would always question the reliability of any tumor marker blood work Obviously, in our case there were other unknown forces in play here which caused the reading to drastically decrease, but yet the cancer was running rampant. All our doctors struggled for an explanation of the correlation between the two, CEA readings and the PET/CT scans.

This was an exceptionally hard, pardon the pun, pill to swallow because the scan just a scant four months ago had been filled with such promise, and the CEA tumor marker readings were promising. Remember, the pathology test for HER/2 had found Mick's to be the type that was not particularly aggressive. But, back to reality—my wife and I looked at each other, stunned beyond belief. Both at the same moment, we turned to the doctor and said, "Let's do the brain again."

In agreement, he being almost as puzzled as we were about the devastating news, he said he would set it up as soon as possible. Explanation from him as to why the reading had dropped so drastically yet we were now faced with a myriad of new locations was difficult; I think even for him this was a shock.

First, I want to be sure everyone knows what a CT or CAT scan is. Medical professional use so many acronyms now you often have to stop and ask, and it's not only doctors and medical people, but everyone you speak with If you don't believe me, just try to read a teenager's text message; they have their own set of acronyms! CATs and CTs are the same thing, meaning "computerized axial tomography." Sometimes they are performed without a contrasting dye and sometimes with. In the case of with, a contrasting agent is injected and this material provides a different look than plain soft tissue because of its ability to reflect the machine's probing rays. These rays are taken in "slices" of the area being looked at and can be three-dimensional.

The pictures turned out by our CAT/CT of the brain, with and without contrast, were anything but a cause for hope. The scan revealed "at least four cerebral masses," none of which could be taken lightly. The first location was in the left cerebellar hemisphere, the area just in front of and above the left ear. It measured 9 mm, a little over a quarter inch. It was already causing some swelling around the area. The next one was in the right cerebral hemisphere, kind of in the middle of this area, but above an area that is called a ventricle. Remember the left eye problem? Hmmm, since the right side of the brain controls the left side of the body, maybe a connection? Let's go to number three tumor— ain't this fun? Imagine it being a picture of your soul mate's brain! The third of these ugly little monsters was located in the top left rear of her brain, very near the skull bone, and it might have been applying pressure on the occipital lobe, where, you guessed it, vision is processed! Now, about number four of these devastating pictures. The technical location was—ready?—"Anterior to the left sylvian fissure." What and where the hell is that, you ask. Well, in plain wording, here goes—first, the sylvian fissure is a dividing membrane that separates parts of the brain. You have one on the right and one on the left. In our pictures, we could see a tumor in front of this membrane, the left one, near the top of her head. Adding insult to injury is the fact that all of these tumor areas are showing swelling, which in medical terms is call edema. The last statement the physician gave was his "impression," which led us to think his feelings were, "What did you expect?" The impression read, "At least four cerebral metastases, **but** this is a woman with breast cancer and previous cerebral metastases." Not much hope in that impression!

As devastated as we were, we managed to compose ourselves and begin investigation as to any treatment options. After consultations with our primary oncologist, the radiation doctor, the breast cancer specialist, and the neurosurgeon it was decided that another scan should be done to assure everyone what we were dealing with. The feeling was if the CAT scan was showing four, a more accurate scan, an MRI, would in all probably confirm more tumors and lesions. Can you believe it? As if the four weren't bad enough, now they're telling us there may be more of these cancer "communities" in her brain! Review here, an MRI, Magnetic Resonance Imaging, scan sends radio waves through an area of the body and measures the response with a computer. This test can also be done with or without a contrasting agent; even without a contrast it is much clearer that the CAT. This was scheduled for February 17, a Sunday, which was good for us since we were going to Baltimore to have it done.

Well, our MRI was, to use the word again, devastating. Technically the report said, "There are multiple new parenchymal (brain) metastases identified, measuring up to 13 mm, involving the bilateral cerebral and cerebellar hemispheres as well as a 5 mm right midbrain lesion and a punctate left potine lesion. There is a new calvarial metastatic lesion within the left frontal bone."

Wow, a lot to absorb, especially through tears as the radiation specialist was telling us he sees "at least thirteen tumors and lesions." First, the measured ones. Thirteen millimeters is a little over half an inch, 5 mm is a little under a quarter inch. The doctors went on to explain that the 13 mm guy was actually applying some pressure on the brain stem; it and the 5 mm tumor were both in precarious locations, and, in all likelihood, neither could be treated. The problem with treatment to either of these was the probability of decreasing quality of life issues; they gave examples of the kind of things that could happen by damage to the surrounding brain tissue. Damage to these areas would in all probability lead to speech and motor function problems, decreased vision or blindness, and, worst of all, a permanent vegetative state or death.

Well, after the devastating news from the brain MRI, we gathered ourselves together, summoned strength from deep within, and began consultation with all our doctors. We first wanted to be sure we had no surgical options, so we contacted the neurosurgeon from the original surgery. After reading the report from the MRI, he let us know that surgery was not an option because of the location and the sheer number of problem areas. Next we consulted the cancer specialists, both our oncologist and the breast cancer specialist. It was their opinion that there were not many choices, as far as medicines go, to treat the conditions in the brain. It seems there is a belief among some doctors that the brain has a "blood barrier," which prevents many medicines from reaching the it, kind of like the brain has its own little protective shield. Some doctors believe this to be true; some do not. Personally, I just question this theory. If cancer meds can't get into the brain, how can a headache medicine stop headache pain, how does an antidepressant medicine reach the neurons in the brain to stop depression, how will an Alzheimer's medicine ever help anyone? The two cancer specialists on our team offered little hope for treatment with medication, and they were of the opinion that all the cancer sites below the neck were not nearly as important as the brain issue. Unless or until we could get a handle on the brain, they thought we should not concern ourselves with treatment for those issues.

After exhausting all hope for treatment with drugs or surgery, we were left with one option: Hello, radiation doctor. Our consultation with him was the first time we heard the word terminal and the phrase "the disease has entered its final stages." Although we both knew the picture was bleak and hope was fading fast, I think actually hearing it struck a blow that is indescribable. He went to say how bleak the picture actually was. Full brain radiation would give her more time, but was not to be misconstrued as a cure. We had heard "full brain radiation" before; we'd already been there, done that. We were surprised to learn it can be done a second time, but the radiation has to be carefully administered because the human brain can only have so much before it turns to mush. It isn't done that often so there are some unknowns, and to top it off, the radiation in and of itself will probably, should one survive, in a couple of years cause tumors of its own.

At this time we asked the question, which I would imagine comes to everyone faced with the word terminal. How long do we have? After all our consultations with all the doctors, it was now left to this poor man, our radiation doctor, to tell us, with no certainty, that without the full brain radiation we might have six to nine weeks. If we elected to do the full brain radiation a second time we could expect six to nine months!

Six to nine weeks? Are you kidding me? was my first thought. *This is the love of my life; we've been together for forty years; she's still young. Barely past fifty-five.* A thousand thoughts came all at once. I had always been her solid foundation, her steady rock throughout this entire cancer story. Now it was all I could do to hold it together and not break down! Remember, this is a lady of whom doctors said you would never know she has cancer unless you look at the pictures, and she still was healthy looking, vibrant, laughing, smiling. She had tolerated all that had been thrown at her for the past two and a half years. The radiation specialist at Baltimore had even remarked how well she had done, going on to tell us that he would normally expect to see these reoccurrences two years ago! She had already become a rarity because it seems that only 2 percent of patients with diagnosis such as the one she was given in 2005 survive this long!

So what do you do? You want to have your loved one as long as possible, but I did not want her to suffer or be in any pain. We, of course, opted to have the full brain radiation again, even given the known side effects of memory loss, eye and vision problems, and maybe even some motor function problems. I think in the back of our minds also was the knowledge that cancer medicines and treatment change rapidly. Who knew what could happen in this field in the next three, six, or nine months?

After this meeting with the radiation doctor we went home and began to absorb all that was happening. I was using every will I had not to break down and fall apart, because I knew this would do her no good. I did find time the next morning, while she was sleeping, and many, many mornings after that, to shed more tears than I thought possible. We have always been spiritual people, content in our belief that there is something after this life. After all, it was this faith that kept us contented in our time of need. We visited a priest; seeing as how we live one block from the church, it wasn't a big trip. We had already approached the subject of death, back in 2005 when this whole chapter of our life started. We knew she had decided to be cremated, but being from a Catholic background, she wanted assurance this was not wrong.

As of late February 2008, we were out of options. Full brain radiation was set to begin again on the February 25, a Monday, and there would be twenty treatments, one every weekday for twenty days. Along with the radiation came the need for another hockey mask mold, and Mick was back on steroids to reduce the swelling caused by the tumors and the swelling induced by the radiation. My wife so despised the steroids that she talked the doctor into waiting to start until she felt she needed them. She managed to hang on for twelve treatments before the headaches became too much to bear, so steroids started slowly, 4 mg a day at first.

Sometimes, I think about the end of February, after a few treatments we were sitting on the steps in the back of our home and this brave, courageous lady turned to me and said, "You know what? I hate that life has done this to us, but I'm not ready to give up yet. I can get busy living or I can get busy dying, and I'm still going to try to be as normal as possible." With that said, she went into the house, got on her walking shoes and said, "Let's go for a walk." We walked the beach, bundled up against the cold, picked up the little shells rolling in the surf, talked about the smell of the sea, the amazingly clear bluest of skies, but neither one of us approached the "C" word during this walk. She seemed to take it all in, enjoying all the little things because we knew there might not be too many more walks on the beach for her.

By the end of treatment number twelve, what little hair that had grown back since 2005—yes, she actually had grown some hair back, albeit skimpy—seemed to disappear. After fifteen treatments the steroids had been increased to 6 mg a day or 2 mg three times a day. This dosage seemed to control her headache and did not interrupt her sleep pattern. As it would turn out, we only had to go through nineteen treatments, Whoopee! The machine broke, and number twenty was canceled.

The treatment ended on March 20, 2008. Mick was showing some fatigue. Her eyes still bothered her, and she was having some balance problems. At this point no one was sure whether they were due to radiation or tumor growth. It now became a waiting game. But Mick wasn't one to pay the waiting game; on March 27 we headed for Florida, again! This Florida trip would be different. She seemed to have less energy, and walking was becoming more and more difficult, as was her balance, and her short-term memory was getting really bad! She loved to go to the street festivals and such, but this time she had difficulty just navigating the rough pavement of Sarasota and the other little areas. Even walking on the beach became difficult because the motion of the surf caused her to be more off balance. Still, she refused to stop and become a "house hermit," as she would put it.

I think this was the time I, along with my brother and sister-in-law, realized this was the beginning of her loss of dignity. That's what metastatic brain cancer often does to its victims. My wife and I had talked of this before and she, being independent, strong willed, and really not dependent on anyone or anything, was apprehensive about entering such a phase of indignation. At first she insisted we only help her to stand, and then she would walk as best she could to where she needed to go. Even more amazing was the fact that she said she wasn't in any pain. Occasionally she would say her leg muscles hurt but I think this was caused by her struggle to continue walking as best she could. Toward the end of this Florida trip we did manage to talk her into getting a cane, a fold up one, that would help her keep her balance and maybe save a tumble!

On this, her last Florida trip, she suddenly got the urge that she would like to try the wig thing again. You remember my words about the first episode regarding a wig; well, why and what suddenly brought this to her desires I'll never know! We visited the shopping mall of Port Charlotte, Florida, along with my brother and his wife. We actually had gone there for dinner, and there was a small wait. As she strolled by the wig shop something attracted her fancy. After much laughing and commenting on different wigs she chose another one, much like the one years ago—you know, the one with real hair! Again the one she chose looked as natural as could be, but she said it had "too much hair." Well, wouldn't you know it; there was a beautician in the mall who was an expert at thinning wigs. Heard this before? Again the wig was thinned, looked as natural as could be, but never to be worn on her little head! I guess I'll make another donation to the breast cancer folks soon.

We returned to our home in Maryland in mid-April, and she continued to take her daily walks, although now they seemed to really tire her out. She really did not have a favorite time of year, but in spring she enjoyed walking on the beach and through the neighborhood to see spring flowers sprouting and the early signs of summer. It seemed now that she seemed to focus on the really simple pleasures—tulips starting to bloom, leaves uncurling on tree branches—it was as if she had made peace with the fact she would never see these earthly things again. Our daily walks continued to get shorter and shorter with each passing day, first around the neighborhood, then down the street—the down the street walks often required me carrying a bag to pick up trash—then they shortened to around the block, and finally by the end of April she could make it only down our driveway and back, a short walk of about a hundred and fifty feet. Our home has five steps to get into, and these five steps really became a struggle by the end of April. She refused to let me pick her up and carry her up the steps. She had always disliked being off her feet. I guess being on her own legs gave her a sense of security. She would struggle to make the steps for a few more days. As the disease continued to disable her, she cried every time I picked her up to move her.

It was becoming more and more difficult for her to be what

she wanted, as normal as possible. I struck up the conversation about a battery scooter to help her be mobile without much assistance from me. At first, she refused my offer to take her to look at them, insisting she wasn't that handicapped. She had now started taking daily walks around inside the house, just to keep exercising. She would walk in a circle from our family room, through the dining room, through the living room, down the hall, and back to where she began. This "walk" was about fifty steps for me, but for her, because she could only take baby steps, it was a lot more. At first, she made the circle with me behind her for assurance that, if she began to wobble, I could steady her. As time progressed, I wound up in front of her, walking backward with her holding my outstretched hands. Even this gave her a great sense of accomplishment to know she still had some independence.

She finally agreed to go look at scooters, because, she said, "Eventually I will need one." We arrived at the dealer and upon entering the showroom, she immediately spied—a cat! This fuzzy fellow was curled on the seat of one of the scooters, and she immediately began to pet him. I think he sensed that she needed to sit, so he moved one scooter over where she could still reach and stroke his back. Well, the scooter he had been lying on was a three-wheeled model. After riding it around the showroom, we thought it was unstable when turning sharply. So she decided she wanted to take the four-wheeled model the cat was now on outside for a test-drive, even though she felt badly about making him move, again. In just a few short minutes the salesman and I turned, and she was completely across the parking lot coming back to us at "rabbit speed." (The scooter has speed setting indicated by a turtle for slow and of course, a rabbit for fast.) The four-wheeled one was her choice, and even though she needed it NOW, she insisted, "It will be there when I need it."

After she had been back on the steroids for a month and a half, the doctors suggested there might be some other reason for her decreasing ability to walk. In an effort to be sure that there wasn't a separate issue effecting her walking ability, they agreed that there was an outside chance there was a tumor on her spine so—let's do a scan—hmmm, haven't had one of those in about, oh, two months! This time it would be an MRI of her "thoracic spine." This is the part of the spine located behind the chest, not quite up to the neck and not quite to the lumbar section at the bottom of the spine. We already knew she had a tumor on the T-9 vertebrae, which did not appear to be compressing the spinal cord. Well, this scan gave credence to fact there were no tumors pressing on the spinal cord but—ready for this?—she now has tumors on her T-2 and T-8 vertebrae and, to top it off, at the T-6 and T-7 location she had a disk pushing sideways—they call it laterally—which was "slightly contacting the cord," but apparently no indications this was cause or reason for her inability to walk. So what do we have? At least three tumors in her spine and a semi-ruptured disk! Yet, to everyone's amazement, she had no back pain to speak of. I was beginning to wonder if this little lady just has a very high tolerance to pain, or maybe the tumor near her brain stem was pinching the pain nerve, if there is such a thing.

It was now mid-May of 2008 and she had lost all ability to walk. Her legs had good strength, which we tested by having her push against me with her legs. She could practically pick me up in the air. Strength was not an issue. But she could not stand without help from me. The problem was that the signal from the brain telling her to put one foot in front of the other did not work. She had relented to allow the scooter in our home. It was a small model, easily disassembled and reassembled. It was so small I could set her on it and ride her into our downstairs bathroom where she could use the potty. She could motor around the whole downstairs pretty easily, although sometimes her eyesight wasn't the best, and she'd hit the wall, make a mark, fold her arms, and then make me drive!

I want to tell of a decision we made back in 2004 when building our home; that decision was now worth its weight in gold. Talk about foresight! We had installed an elevator! Yeah, a residential type which was big enough for her scooter to fit in. We first thought about it not because we thought she would have cancer again and, oh, we might have to get a scooter upstairs. The thought was maybe there would be a time when her elderly mom might have to live with us, and this would make her stays more pleasant. This miracle decision we made in 2004 was now a lifesaver. Mick was able to go up to our bedroom, stay in her own bed, and even use her own bathroom. I would lift her into her scooter downstairs, drive it into the elevator, and proceed to go upstairs. What a convenience.

As time passed, she became more dependent upon her scooter. I built a ramp down our back steps that enabled her to get to ground level. This gave her access to the outdoors, freedom from being cooped up. She would ride around the block, point out trash for me to pick up, and she could even go into the church. She especially enjoyed looking at the different yards; even though she had run and walked by them many times, there was still a new discovery with every ride. She now even enjoyed the grocery store. Before the inability to walk set in she would zip through the stores as quickly as possible, get what we needed, and get out. Now she stopped at different products, read labels, and fussed about the prices. She even had a little basket where she could carry all her goodies!

Although she became more dependent on the scooter, it was in a way a loss of dignity. She was still dependent on me to get her onto it and off of it. It seems as if the disease disabled her starting from the feet upward. And with the loss of each process came a little more indignation. Each morning I would greet her as she woke and of course after discussion about how she felt, I would pick her up and set her onto her scooter to begin her day.

One particular morning I pulled back the covers and slid my arms behind her shoulders and under her knees. Then, turning to sit her on the cart, I realized she felt very heavy and resistant. I turned to see that she had clutched in her little hands the comforter, blanket, and sheet. I told her, "Honey, you have to let go of something." She then, much to my relief, turned loose of the bed linens and started to laugh, stating it was a mystery to her why she clutched so tightly to the covers. She said maybe she had become like the Snoopy character, the one that needed a security blanket. It did my heart good to hear her laugh; she stayed that way till the end, always a ready smile for everyone.

Another indignation she suffered through was being dependent on me to get her into and out of the bathtub. The assistance I gave her was simple at first; I would help her into the tub and then leave her to soak and enjoy her bath. As it became more evident she needed help to get in and out of the tub, I always made sure she had her cell phone near her. I remember one time in particular I left her in the tub and told her to call and I'd be back to help her. After what seemed like an hour, I realized I had not heard from her. I went up to the bathroom and found her sitting in an empty tub crying. I asked, "Why didn't you call?"

She looked at me with tears in her eyes and said, "I couldn't remember any number to call." Even though we had been married for almost thirty-six years and had enjoyed baths, showers, and loving moments, this somehow was different for her, a complete loss of independence. Baths were a particularly rough time. It seemed after soaking and washing in the warm water she lost all ability to stand or move. I didn't know if there was a disease connection or if the stress of having to struggle to stand took a toll on her. I would have to pick her up from the tub, sit her on a stool, dry her off, and then dress her, after which I would carry her to the bed where she would rest for ten to fifteen minutes and then she could stand and turn onto her scooter.

As late May approached her eyesight had gotten to the point where she had a lot of double vision and what she called "gray vision," an inability to see colors. This eye problem, coupled with the radiation to her brain and the tumor location, made concentration difficult. She was still involved in the small consulting work she had been doing, but now I had to read most of it to her and then take dictation. Her attention span was limited to about an hour on any one thing, and then she would get fatigued and lose concentration. Her eyesight presented a problem with the scooter operation also. She had trouble with depth perception and began to run into things, or she was unable to hold the scooter in a straight line. Along with this came more dependence on me. Now I had to be her driver, too. Nothing I had to do for her caused me any difficulty or ambiguous feelings; I was happy and proud to care for the one I loved.

In late May, with all the increasing difficulty she was having, we began to question whether the second round of full brain radiation had any effect at all. We requested another MRI of the brain, just to answer this question. It seems the radiation doctor was a little hesitant. His reasoning was that no matter what the results of an MRI there was little he could do with the remaining brain cancer.

The MRI was done on May 22, 2008, and the results were helpful in relieving our concerns about whether the radiation had been a failed attempt at helping a dire situation. The radiation had in fact decreased tumors in the cerebellar and cerebral regions, but—seems as if there's always a "but" with these scans—the tumor in the periventricular location had increased in size. I know, I know, where and what is a periventricular location?

I now know quiet a bit about the brain, probably more than anyone wants or needs to know unless they're confronted with illness connected with this organ. It seems that the periventricular area is actually a structure in the brain called the—ready?—hypothalamus, a little part of the brain about the size of an almond that provides a link to the nervous system. Its location is near the pituitary gland and precariously close to the brain stem. It seems this little guy controls, hum, let's see, body temperature—maybe that's why she's cold in seventy degree weather; hunger—maybe that's why her appetite is decreasing; thirst—maybe this is why her water intake has decreased; fatigue—well, she is really tired a lot; and anger—and I was blaming this on radiation effects—how silly of me. Even more revealing, it affects responses to light and vision.

This scan also revealed that the tumor in her left frontal area still persisted and also had increased activity. So, the diagnosis was some tumor activity has slowed, but the most deadly ones continued and would continue to contribute to her demise, especially the one at the brain stem—as stated before, a location no one wishes to enter. The advice we were given was to stay the course with the steroids to prevent swelling and pressure and to make contact with the hospice people in our area. We had already discussed this scenario, not so much for everyday care but for medical checks and such that could be done without a trip to the doctor's office.

I would imagine anyone that has had to talk about his or her demise found it difficult. Beginning in February with the diagnosis of terminal, she and I found it less upsetting with each talk. She knew she wanted to discuss our past, my future, my health problems, and a memorial for her, in that order.

She had always been a realist, judging each situation intelligently and sorting through the why and wherefores. So it came as no surprise to me that she was able to discuss this openly and without a lot of sadness or regret. We first discussed, over a period of days and weeks, the life we had lived together and our disappointments and accomplishments, the pride we had in each other, and some of the things we both considered amazing that we were able to see through till the end. She was extremely proud that we had never lived in a home we did not build. She was proud of our ability to maintain two homes for many years of our lives, one of which was our dream beach house, which became a reality in 1982. I think she was also proud of her career and the fact that she got to travel the world, many trips with me by her side. I think her pride in her career came from the fact that she had chosen not to attend college and to begin at the very bottom government entry level, and to enjoy her job until retirement. She was basically a shy girl, not comfortable in a public forum, yet she was able to overcome this and travel and conduct meetings and conferences with her colleagues, co-workers, and business associates. Although she never said it, and she never would, I could tell her career was a proud achievement for her.

One of the greatest disappointments for her was early in our marriage, in 1979; she had a tough time with her feelings and where she was in her life. She knew then and she recalled now how heartbroken I was when she thought there was more to life than she was experiencing. I probably had a hand in this as I worked a lot, my regular job, then, till late in the evenings on most Saturdays, I would be gone doing electrical work somewhere. I realized, later, when we discussed this, that she had became lonely. After all, she wasn't quite twenty when we were married, very young, even in the 1970s. When this initially happened, even as heartbroken as I was, I thought it wise not to interfere with her happiness or decision as to where she wanted to head. I actually left for a while so she could decide her future. We had no doubts about my future; I made it clear I wanted her for eternity! She had the opportunity, without outside inference, to make a decision that made me the happiest and luckiest guy in the world; she made the decision to stay with me for what would turn out to be forever for her.

As for other disappointments, there weren't any significant enough to remember. The one subject we had conversations about earlier in our marriage, the thought of a family, was not a source of disappointment for her at all. She had no regrets about not being a mother. We have numerous nieces and nephews; she loved them immensely, but was always happy they could go home with someone else. Looking back now, she remarked that we probably would not have had the many opportunities we did experience had there been children—not that she said this selfishly, but since we both had gotten involved with careers very early, the family issue took a backseat. She always had admiration for the women who could juggle careers and motherhood. We remembered when my brother's twins were born in 1970 we would often travel and go to shopping malls with them. We would take one twin, and they would take the other. We sometimes liked to play games with the people that approached. They would say, "Oh, look, twins!" We would joke saying, "They're not twins, that one is their son and this one is ours." The people would remark how uncanny it was the boys looked so much alike; sometimes we told them the facts, sometimes we didn't.

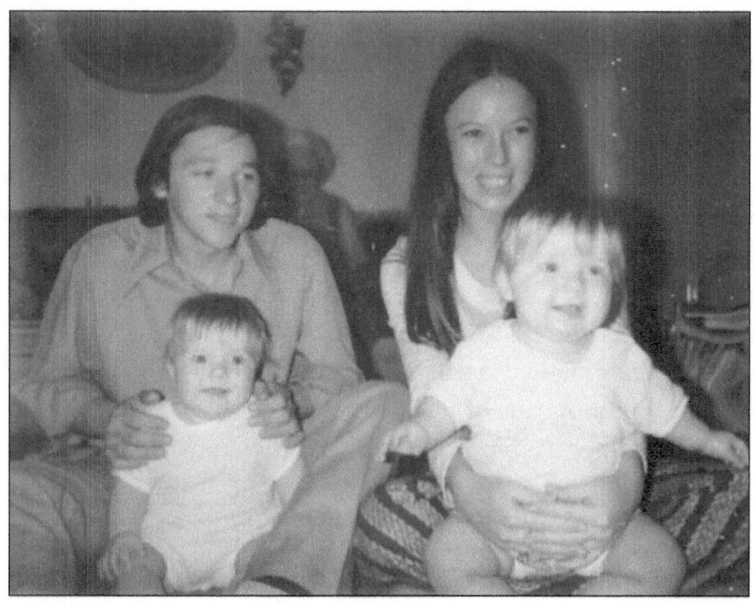

My wife to be and I with brother's twins, 1971

We shared the memory of my little adventure into the world of drag racing. In the early 1990s, four of my brothers and some friends were involved in the sport and they encouraged, me to spend a few Saturdays at the local drag strip. After attending and watching several races with them, I thought I would like to participate, to bond with my family, as that seemed more fun than watching. I converted Mick's car, one she had for about thirteen years, into a weekend race car. We bought her another car to replace this older one; although it wasn't a new car it was fast—remember, this is the lady who as a young gal needed a car to "get out of the way of a tractor trailer." We attended many weekend races around the area for several years, and then we realized the sport was cutting into our weekends at the beach, something we both enjoyed. Then, as fate would have it, the 1996 diagnosis of breast cancer happened. With that issue and our love for the beach, I ended my drag racing career. Here and now during this talk I learned I had broken her heart when I took "her favorite car" and turned it into a race car.

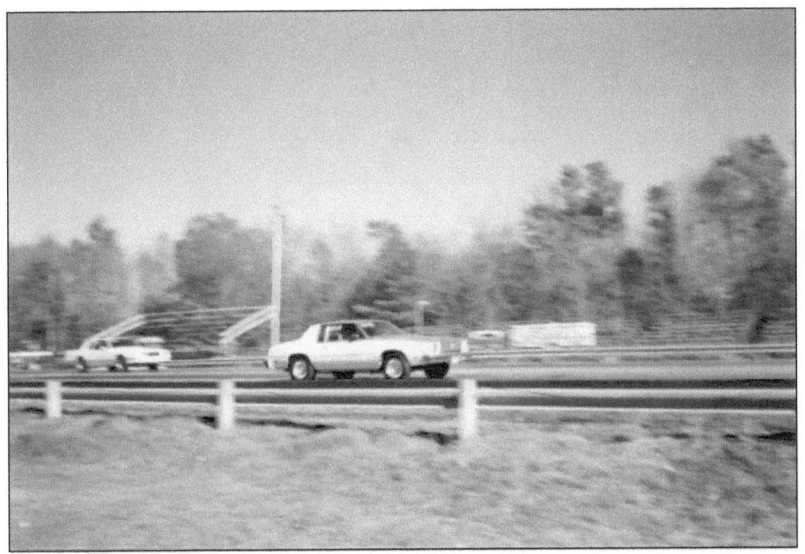

Her favorite car, my race car

Another thing she was secretly proud of was her athleticism, her running, racquetball skills, tennis, and, not least of all, her softball career; she had played on various leagues for more than fifteen years. Her softball career ended when the government office she worked for changed location and the new facility did not allow beer. That did it! She retired from organized softball. As far as the running thing, this became another thing she did with a passion. She did this for more than twenty years. She was proud of all the countries and places where she had the opportunity to run: almost all of the Caribbean Islands, Mexico, Athens, Hawaii, Guam, and many, many cities across the United States. If she missed running at lunch I usually had to suffer through a three to six miler in the evening. She enticed me to join her more times than I like to say! I was never the dedicated runner she was, but I ran with her on many occasions when we traveled. I never lasted the twenty or so years she did. I was kind of a run-when-I-felt-like-it guy, unless she offered me fringe benefits to run with her!

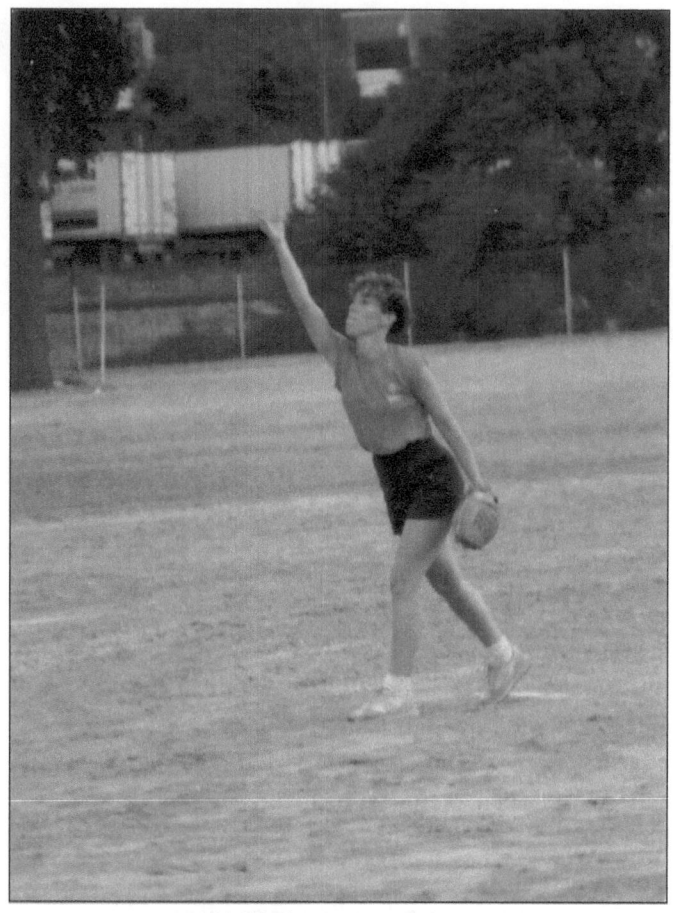

Softball player extraordinaire

I remembered her dedication to running: This one cold January day in the mideighties, we were at our beach house when she decided to go for a run since it was "sunny." Please, it was, like, twenty degrees outside with a northeast wind howling about twenty miles an hour! She decided she would only run south and instructed me to come pick her up in about an hour. I thought to myself, *This woman's nuts!* She put on umpteen layers of clothes, long johns, tights, sweatpants, double socks, sweatshirt, scarf, and earmuffs, and—oh yeah—a bandana over her mouth to "keep from freezing her lungs!" Well, I waited about a half hour and headed south on the coastal highway. About three miles down the highway I spotted her. She was still going. I did a U-turn, opened the door, and in she scampered. She looked worse than Jesse James with a frozen bandana! The bandana was so stiff with frozen condensation that it weighed a ton! I told her she would be lucky if she didn't get a stiff neck from holding her head up with weight of that bandana hanging on her face! But dedicated she was and this was normal for her. We chuckled about this memory, and then our thoughts turned to sadness because now she could not even stand.

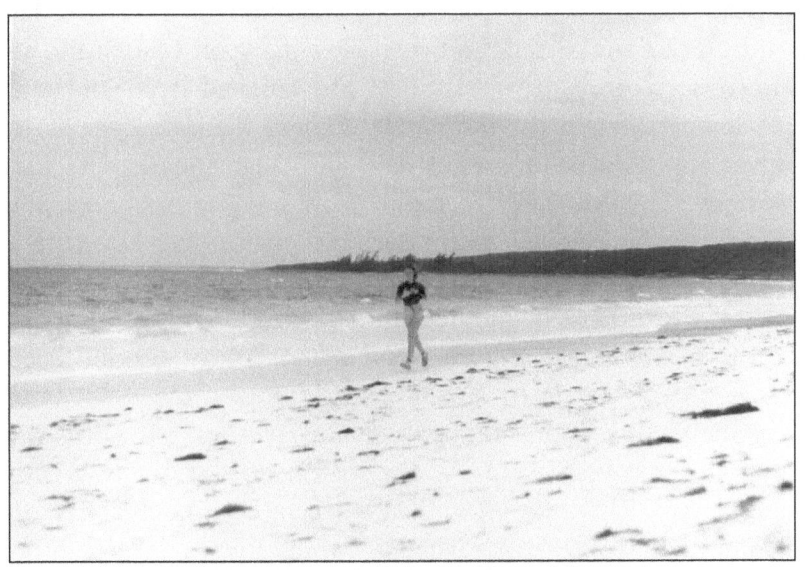

Running on a Bahamas beach, 1979

She had a way of being very serious with me, yet tricking me. We recalled how recently, on one of our trips to Florida, she had conned me into going shopping with her, and as my brother will attest, shopping with my wife or my sister-in-law can turn into an all-day affair. There was a department store I was not familiar with that she wished to shop in. She had dragged me all around that day; I was through with shopping, but she said while she

looked I could go through the "tool" department, "just like Sears."
Well, I relented, like most guys, um tools!. This store didn't have
a tool department, and they were insulted when I tried to find it.
Mick was hysterical to think she had actually tricked me again!
Now, here, talking about our life and her death, and what it had
been and was going to be, she again laughed till she cried. What
bravery, facing a death sentence and still being able to block it
out and laugh, again being, "as normal as possible."

Another memory she brought to our talks was about her
inability to remember holidays, birthdays, and anniversaries;
sure, she knew the major ones, Christmas and Thanksgiving!
We laughed about how one year she had bought me a birthday
card on our anniversary and then later that year bought me an
anniversary card on my birthday! She laughed it off and said
it was the thought that counted. When I reminded her of an
upcoming holiday or special day, she'd just remark, "It's just
another day." This inspired me to write her another poem; she
was the inspiration for many poems over our years together. I
knew she never kept them all so I was surprised to find in her
dresser a few weeks before her death an envelope containing five
of the poems I had written her. I asked, "Why did you keep
these?"

She simply said, "Those were my favorites." The five she
kept all those years were "As Twenty Passes," for our twentieth
anniversary, "Just Another Day," which I wrote for her on
Valentine's Day 1995, "Beachgoer," which I wrote for her forty-
third birthday, "Tied," which I wrote for her on our twenty-fifth
anniversary, and "After Three Decades," a thirty-first anniversary
poem.

Our love has stood the test of time
Since we became valentines
Through triumphs and heartaches
Seeing other lovers, so fake.
I wanted you then, I want you now,
Stay my valentine; we'll make it somehow
Until we grow old I'll always care
My heart, my soul and my feelings I'll share.
Our love is special and in the passing time
We'll be even more glad we became valentines
I sometimes think and wonder where,
If we weren't valentines would we still care?
I know you'll think and say, it's just another day,
Remembering special days was not your way
But days are what we have, Valentine,
Stay—till the end of time!

Another of the "hard talks" we had wasn't about her, our past, or memories. The talk was about my future and me. In my view, I think she was overly concerned about my health and the conditions I mentioned previously in this story. This kind of talk was extremely difficult for me, talking about the future without her.

As we talked about my future she was insistent that I do whatever made me find happiness, be it travel, writing, or building, or even falling in love again. She made it clear that I should grieve as long as I needed but that I shouldn't let grief stand in the way of happiness and moving forward. She said that even though we were supposed to "grow old together," it was not going to happen and I should not let my heart "die with her," because, she said, "You're not old." She told me I should find someone to grow old with. She knew the guilt I would feel about loving again, but she insisted I should not feel that way because I had given her my heart for forty years, until her forever came, and I still had so much to give that I shouldn't keep my heart hidden. These kinds of talks often became so emotional for me that I had to excuse myself and leave the room for fear of breaking down in front of her.

Our talks were not all about memories; we had to discuss the subject of her funeral, burial, and memorial. We had already gotten assurance from the Catholic priest that cremation was not considered a sin. This had been her desire for some time, and she still felt strongly about it. On one of our visits to the priest, he had given us a small book with prayers that were sometimes said at funerals and memorials. Over the next few weeks, she read every prayer, shared some with me, and eventually chose her own funeral prayers. There were three of them, not long ones, because she said she didn't want to keep people sitting in the funeral home for hours! She also asked at this time for me to do something that turned out to be one of the hardest things I have ever written. She asked that I write her eulogy, or a remembrance poem, as I call them. I had written remembrance poems and had a card done for other relatives and friends that had passed, and she liked this idea. I told her I would do my best—I mean, come on, how do you write a thing of that nature for the person that is your life?

Also, she had found on the Internet a few years ago something called eternal reefs. I suspect because of her love for the sea and all things connected to it she was probably looking for something to buy to decorate our home. At any rate, she had kept this folder in her file, and she brought it to me and said, "Remember this?" I told her I did and asked her if she still thought that was what she wanted for herself. She went on to tell me this was what she wanted and that she wanted her memorial to be part of the manmade reef off the coast right here in our little town.

For those of you who are wondering what an "eternal reef" is, let me explain. About ten years ago this guy in Florida was working with the federal government to restore reefs that were disappearing for whatever reason. Well, it seems he had a father-in-law who gave him a lightbulb moment by asking that his cremated remains be "put in one of those reef things." The process goes like this: Your loved one is cremated, the ashes are then put in the concrete going into a mold to make a manmade reef. The reef kind of looks like an igloo with holes in it. Then the memorial reef is placed in several permitted locations around different coastlines. You get to have hands-on participation in the casting process! This was her choice and her desire because, as she told me, "I don't want to be a rock sticking out of the ground that people visit for a while, then after a few years they have trouble even remembering where it is." Plus, as she put it, God's creatures in the sea need a place to hide and rest, and the coral that grows on the reef is more beautiful than most flowers. Like I said, a lady that loved the sea and all things associated with it.

There were many of these hard talks over the last months of her life. I call them hard talks because sometimes they were so emotional we both would cry and wish this were not happening. I sometimes, trying to be her rock of support, would have to go outside and break down after we had a talk; it was so hard coming to the realization that "till death do we part" was right here. I will always have admiration for the way she was able to handle her date with destiny, and I only pray God gives me the same strength.

Our talks were interrupted in early May by a memorial for her cousin who had passed away in January. Her son had elected to have a party of remembrance for his mom close to her birthday, May 3. Even though this required us to travel a hundred and sixty miles or so, Mick insisted on attending. I know this was especially hard on her to know that she would soon be the cause for something such as this. The trip seemed especially long to her because the tumors had robbed her of any sense of time. What was actually a three-hour trip seemed like days to her. At the memorial she was her usual self, smiling and laughing and getting teased about the adventures she and her cousin had shared. Many people did not realize nor could they fathom that she had only months to live. She never mentioned it to them; they only learned of the conditions when they questioned me as to why she could not walk. This was the way she had been all her life, quiet and unassuming, never wanting to be the center of attention.

I will be eternally grateful for the last months of her life, and, as hard as it was and is to let go, we had a long time to say good-bye. I have feelings for those whose life comes to an end suddenly; their families and friends are completely caught off guard and sometimes have a hard time coming to grips with the sudden death of a loved one. There probably was something they needed to say to that person. On the same day that my wife passed away, a truck driver ran off a bridge and died on his way to deliver a load. He wasn't even supposed to be driving that day; he had volunteered. I'm sure he left his home saying good-bye to his family, and they surely did not know this was a final good-bye. So, thank God her passing was not sudden and unexpected, and she managed to keep her faculties about her till the very end.

We had come to be dependent on her scooter for aid in moving her, and as the tumors became more pronounced, more indignation came our way. The next indignation she was to suffer was kind of due to two things. She had continued to despise the steroids. They made sleep a problem and they swelled her little face. So in late May we decide to give a try at getting off them so maybe she could rest better, and she would surely feel better if her cheeks didn't look like they belonged on a chipmunk! The doctors agreed and said we should not stop altogether; they had to be tapered down by lessening the dosage a little every few days. We took our time, and by June 6, 2008, we had ended the steroids, albeit slowly.

Well, as it turns out, we needed the steroids more than we realized because the following week she really crashed, and another unexpected issue began and never went away. On June 13 some friends came in from Alabama, and she wanted to meet them at a casino near our home. She loved to play the slot machines, and she had her own little ideas and thoughts about why people did or did not win. She never won much to speak of; she was a penny and nickel warrior. After retirement we would go once or twice a month. A couple of her little tidbits I'll share with you. She always insisted we never go play on a Sunday. Why? Because the casinos were all trying to recoup their losses from Friday and Saturday! She also said you should never leave your player's card in all the time because the casino would know you were a loser. If you continued to lose they knew they had a sucker. Another rule was don't play before six o'clock in the evening. I never did get the reason for that one. I won more often than she did; of course I played a little higher stakes, but she had this uncanny ability, a sixth sense, if you would, to know when I had won. Just about the time I would be getting my payout, I would turn around and there she'd be, holding out her hand and saying, "Can we play longer?" One of our friends who often went with us, usually hung with her because he also was a penny and nickel warrior. He told me they would be in the middle of some "hot machines," and she would suddenly tell him, "Ray's getting paid." Suddenly her machine wasn't so hot; she would cash out and proceed to cruise the casino to find me or she would call me on the cell phone! Memories are priceless!

On the way to the casino, which was about an hour's drive away, Mick began to be rather lethargic and kind of out of sorts. By the time we reached our destination she was unable even to move her legs to turn for her scooter, and she acted like she wasn't sure where she was. We met our friends; she seemed to recognize them but seemed still to be having a hard time grasping reality. I decided it best to check into our room and see if she just needed rest.

The situation worsened, and she was unable to control her bladder. By the time I lifted her onto the bed, we realized there was a problem. I immediately called our doctor; even though it was after seven, I did not hesitate to call. He had always called back when we needed him. He did not let us down; he returned the call promptly, and after I briefed him on the conditions he said we must get back on the steroids, NOW! He instructed me to begin with 8 mg now and another eight at midnight, followed by at least 12 mg the next day. This was not the first time we had tried to get off the steroids; about a month before we had done the same routine—bring her off them slowly—but that time wasn't pleasant either. About two days after stopping she became violently ill, throwing up for what seemed to be hours. So with these two episodes it was quite apparent that the swelling of the area near the brain stem and in her left frontal lobe needed to be controlled with the steroid.

The incident of the June 13 was the beginning of another loss of dignity for her. Not only had her eyesight continued to fail, along with short-term memory and sense of time, nor could she control her emotions—anger, sadness, and such—plus she could not walk, and now she could not control her bladder.

Wetting herself became a constant thing to deal with and with it came the dreaded "granny pants," Depends undergarments. The disease had now progressed to a point where it was difficult for her to even stand, so we devised a method for her to put her arms around my neck. I would stand her up with her feet on top of mine, and I would rotate around so she could sit onto her Porta-Potty. Yet with all these things beginning to accumulate, she still insisted on moving about as best she could. She even wanted to go to the flea market in Brimfield one more time. We decide to go in early July.

The week of July 7, 2008, approached, and she was very apprehensive about the trip, with all the problems she was having, plus the fact she was getting weaker in her arms. Just sliding across a car seat was problematic. I assured her that I would make the trip as comfortable as possible, that a friend and I would not let her down. After all the anxieties she managed to make the trip, and she even found a few things to her liking, some very old prints of jellyfish, a hand woven wicker urn, and an old ship model. Again, for her the trip was an eternity, for her sense of time was completely out of whack. We had to keep reassuring her that we had not taken a wrong route and that we would arrive in due time.

The return trip was even more of a nightmare as we ran into dreadful traffic on the Jersey turnpike. What should have been a seven-hour journey quickly turned into a ten hour one! By the time we arrived in our driveway she was completely exhausted, but I do not know who was the most proud, she or I. I was proud of her for remaining true to her creed of being as normal as possible, and she was proud that she had been able to go one last time. She was still living and viable, and able to enjoy something she had loved. She was so exhausted she could not slide herself across the seat to exit the truck. I had to lift her out and place her onto her scooter to take her inside. As soon as I placed her onto our couch she did not even wait to look at her things; she was asleep within minutes. What a courageous lady, brave to a fault!

It was now July 12, and she was exhibiting signs of weakness and a loss of appetite, in addition to all the other things I mentioned before. The loss of appetite was new as she had always maintained a steady diet and had lost very little weight through this whole ordeal; she was still about a hundred and twenty pounds.

Even with all the problems she had experienced on the trip to Brimfield, she still insisted on Monday, July 14, to go to a framing shop about thirty miles away to select a frame and matting for her antique prints and to help me pick out framing for some watercolor paintings I had purchased. She made the trip to the shop, but inasmuch as her eyesight was very poor, I had to describe colors to her. She was able to see some things by closing one eye to stop the double vision. There would be one more auto ride after this, to our doctor's office for what would be the last visit to him, on July 21, 2008.

We had already made contact with hospice, and for the past few weeks a nurse had been coming to check vitals. On this visit the doctor did his usual check but paid close attention to her feet, raising one up to show me a little swelling around the ankles. After the routine checks—her weight, blood pressure, and temperature—he told us we need not struggle for another appointment as he could get the vitals he needed from the hospice nurse. However, this time he ended the appointment with something he had never done before with my wife. He asked her for a hug. I think he knew then the end was very near.

The next two weeks went by uneventfully; she continued to get up every morning, I would pick her up, put her on her scooter, take her into the bath, she'd wash her face, brush her teeth, and she would put on her face cream. I would drive her to the elevator and go downstairs through our kitchen, but now she had stopped checking out what was there to eat. She even had a hard time making herself want coffee. She would watch some things on TV, and then she usually wanted to go out back and just sit on the porch, but she wanted to be covered with a blanket even though this was early August. Her brain had lost its ability to control her body temperature. She became more and more fatigued, and her daily naps became more necessary.

On the morning of Sunday, August 3, 2008, I came up after

she had rung her bell. I had set up a wireless doorbell so she just had to push the button and I would come to her aid. In the past two weeks she often rang the bell and I would rush upstairs, only to find out she just wanted me there by her side. I would stay by her side until she'd fall asleep for her nap. This particular morning was different. She asked me not to take her downstairs; she was just too tired. I asked if she cared for any breakfast, and she said she'd like a scrambled egg. I went down and prepared the egg, cut it up for her, and went back upstairs. I set her upright with her pillows, and she picked up the fork, but she did not have the coordination to find her mouth. Her arms were finally letting her down, along with all the other things that were letting her down. This was the final indignation she could bear; she looked at me and said, "You shouldn't have to do this," and with that she never ate again.

The tumors were also taking away her voice, and her eyes were really affected by any kind of light. She refused to allow the draperies to be closed all day, so I had to open them ever so slightly so she could sense the day and night. Her voice continued to deteriorate to nothing more than a whisper, although we would still lie side by side with my ear close to her face and talk about our life together. She had lost the ability to turn onto her side so I would help her turn over to the side she desired and then put a pillow behind her to hold her there. On the evening of Wednesday, August 6, she asked to be turned onto her left side. I got out of bed, went to her side, and did as she asked. As we lay talking she suddenly found the strength to put her right arm and hand across me. She patted my chest three times and said, "You're gonna be okay." Those were the last words she ever spoke.

After the loss of her voice she continued to know friends were visiting, even smiling her beautiful little crooked smile when someone talked of a fond memory. There were many neighbors, family, and friends from her childhood who came to visit over the next few days, and they all shared their memories and suffered their grief and pain silently in her presence. On Saturday, August 9, at about 3:30 AM, the love of my life, my world it seemed, lapsed into a coma, and thirty hours later, with my brother and I each holding a hand, God ended her cancer war.

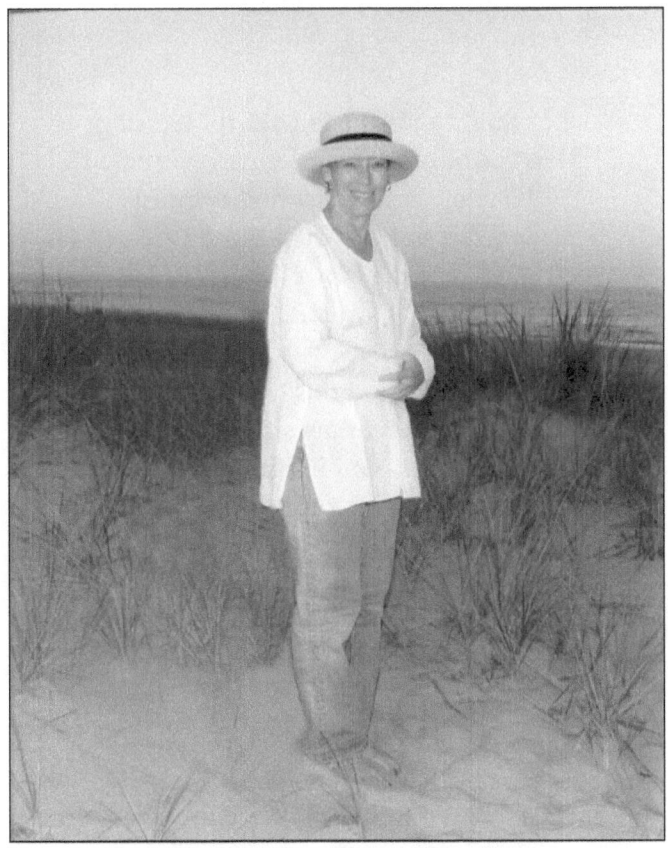

Her last picture, September of 2007

A Caregiver's Prayer

My Lord, on this day I give thanks
Thanks for giving me the guidance
Skills and patience to help my
Loved one cope with the daily battles
Against a raging disease.

My Lord, on this day I pray
That you have given me the strength
All that I needed to do my best
And all that I could have done
To ease their burden.

My Lord, on this day I ask for blessing
Bless the one whose suffering I witnessed
Bless me that I may find comfort
Comfort in knowing I did my best
For the battle is over
My job is done.

My Lord, on this day I pray
I pray for forgiveness of my sin and shortcomings
May they be few and insignificant, so that
I may be reunited with the one I cared for
In Heaven's glory

Amen

═══ EULOGY POEM ═══

I did write her that eulogy poem and made a card for everyone to
have from her memorial; she never got to read it. It's followed by
her three favorites, the ones I found and asked about.

So now it has come to this,
Two score and more from childhood bliss,
This angel, our angel so filled with love
Ascends to Heaven, on wings of the purest of doves.

For all of us she touched, loved, or cared about,
Through all our sadness, remember, she wouldn't pout,
Remember her laughing eyes, her ready smile,
For she's in Heaven, we'll see her in awhile.

We don't know if she had a plan for life,
She became a friend, a companion, a wife,
She started very young on life's winding road,
She worked, she traveled, she'd carry your load.

Her travels through life, to places some never see,
But she always returned, excited, just to be,
A friend, a companion to us, you and me,
So now Heaven's home, her heart held the key.

Sometimes frustrated when life didn't go her way,
She cared deeply, she wanted her say,
Then when all was said and done,
She'd crumble for fear of hurting someone.

Some of us were close, some were not,
But all she touched will miss her, a lot,
And all should remember she would console
Us in our grief, which lies deep in our souls.

I know It's been said on many a line,
She was special, one of a kind,
But believe these words, her companions and friends,
Heaven's roads she'll learn, every crook, every bend.

This special lady with the biggest of hearts,
Looked into our lives and became a part
Of our life's journeys, each and everyone,
Let us remember a life, bright as the sun.

As Twenty Passes

Some twenty years ago today
We set out on our way
A journey together we began
Two hearts as one, hand in hand.

When our marriage was fresh and new
We were young and facing a sky of blue
And I think we both realized
That blue wouldn't always be the sky.

As years passed and life would get us down
Neither was afraid to be the fool, the clown.
We both felt if times were tough and you can smile
There's a warm love, it will last a long while.

Neither of our hearts burned like a wild flame
We were always equal, practically the same
For if one loves more than the other
Life's little secrets, they're harder to discover.

As we grew and began to discover
The joys of life, and each other,
We'd talk, laugh, smile, and love and we're finding
Our love grows and becomes the strongest of bindings.

We play, we travel, we discover
Perhaps there was a sign to be lovers,
In going through the months and years
We've had the same joys, the same fears.

I was never afraid to let you be you
And with me being me, we stuck like glue.
Being married to you sure is nice,
Never a thing of sacrifice.

We've been through good times, sad times, bad times
And we've come through each with good signs.
This union of two hearts, yours mine, mine yours
We could walk in and out of all the doors.

So, in hope for the future, let me say
I hope to love you each and every day
And for the next twenty years and more,
Here's to knowing you and I will dance on the same floor.

═ Tied ═

For oh so long our hearts have been tied
Times of joy, love, laughter, and we've cried
We committed to each other so young
Who could have predicted what had begun.

Long ago in our small world
We began this journey; my, how it's unfurled
We seem to have weathered the times
Both of us ever heeding the signs.

Neither of us ever wanted to be some other place
Both of us contented with a familiar face.
So it is that we will go on, forever
These two hearts being untied; never.

I look forward to future years
Knowing you'll be there; no fears.
Together we will always stay
Cause hearts intended it that way.

So, please my angel, wear this token
Close to your heart and believe these words I've spoken
Cause you and I are forever tied
Form our hearts we will never hide.

My love for you is not stored on a shelf
I love you more than life itself
I love you more than life itself
I love you more than------------!

=== AFTER THREE DECADES ===

It doesn't really seem more than three decades ago
We really thought life would go slow
But here we are at retirement's door
I know the future holds so much more.

You've shared my dreams, our passions
We saw a lot go, in and out of fashion
Our life together will go on
Till we meet on a Heaven's dawn.

We've worked together to build our homes and our life,
I am happy and content, with you, my wife,
As we make this turn in the road
I am thankful you'll share the load.

And many years down the road, should we make it
To heaven's gate, our way will be lit,
And if I wanted to, and could, rearrange the stars
I'd only have to look, there you are.

I want to say with great pleasure I was able to grant her every wish regarding her memorials. We had discussed during our hard talks her desires and wishes. She wanted to be cremated and her memorials to become an eternal reef off the coast of Ocean City, Maryland. I can understand her wish and desire to do this because of her love for the sea.

As if I needed more signs that this was the right thing to do, upon receiving her ashes the eternal reef foundries contacted me and asked if I were going to participate in the casting. Are you kidding? I would not have missed it for the world! They then proceeded to tell me the casting date would be Monday, September 8, 2008. You see, this was to be her fifty-sixth birthday! This reinforced my feelings that this was meant to be—the fact that she had chosen something like this that very few people realized was out there as her final memorial, and then that it was to be cast on her birthday. It was the last, the best, and the only possible birthday gift I could give her.

She had chosen three prayers and had discussed with me her desire to have no pictures at the services. She was never one to want her picture taken, even though she was very photogenic, not to mention beautiful. It was a phobia she developed early on in life, I can't tell you why. Well, this is where I told her a little white lie. I agreed, reluctantly, and seeing my disappointment, she relented and said I could have one picture.

I took advantage of her relenting, and I did have only one picture—one of every phase of her life.

After the casting and delivery of her memorial reef there was a dockside ceremony, and the following day a trip four miles off the coast to set it with the community of reefs. Her memorial is located at the coordinates of 38*16.658N—75*01.582W. The company allowed me to put a little verse on the brass identification plaque; it reads:

"Let all god's creatures that pass here find warmth from the soul within."

As for me I'm "gonna be okay," her last words, and I will try to be "as normal as possible." As with everyone who has lost a part of themselves in the loss of a loved one, it's been said to me a million times that time makes it easier to take. Your anger at God will lessen, but the memories are always there.

══ Acknowledgments ══

I wish to express the deepest gratitude and thanks to the many doctors, nurses, and medical people who, in the course of our battle with this disease, treated my wife not as a number or just another patient but as a real person with real feelings and fears. I also wish to express thanks to my family for allowing my wife to be part of their lives from the very beginning until the end, especially those who opened their homes and made us feel welcome. To the many friends that were there for her lifetime, thanks. To her boss for his understanding and dealing with her for so many years, she enjoyed your companionship.

I wish to thank God for giving me his angel for forty years, for giving me strength in my hour of need, for giving me courage to go on without her, and for helping me continue to be *"as normal as possible."*